S.E. WEAVER
905 MAIN AVE.
BROWNWOOD, TEXAS 76801

THE PRUDENT USE OF MEDICINES

TIME LIFE ®
BOOKS

Other Publications:

CLASSICS OF THE OLD WEST
THE EPIC OF FLIGHT
THE GOOD COOK
THE SEAFARERS
THE ENCYCLOPEDIA OF COLLECTIBLES
THE GREAT CITIES
WORLD WAR II
HOME REPAIR AND IMPROVEMENT
THE WORLD'S WILD PLACES
THE TIME-LIFE LIBRARY OF BOATING
HUMAN BEHAVIOR
THE ART OF SEWING
THE OLD WEST
THE EMERGENCE OF MAN
THE AMERICAN WILDERNESS
THE TIME-LIFE ENCYCLOPEDIA OF GARDENING
LIFE LIBRARY OF PHOTOGRAPHY
THIS FABULOUS CENTURY
FOODS OF THE WORLD
TIME-LIFE LIBRARY OF AMERICA
TIME-LIFE LIBRARY OF ART
GREAT AGES OF MAN
LIFE SCIENCE LIBRARY
THE LIFE HISTORY OF THE UNITED STATES
TIME READING PROGRAM
LIFE NATURE LIBRARY
LIFE WORLD LIBRARY

FAMILY LIBRARY:
HOW THINGS WORK IN YOUR HOME
THE TIME-LIFE BOOK OF THE FAMILY CAR
THE TIME-LIFE FAMILY LEGAL GUIDE
THE TIME-LIFE BOOK OF FAMILY FINANCE

*This volume is one of a series designed to familiarize readers
with the latest advances in medical science and to guide them in
maintaining their own health and fitness.*

THE PRUDENT USE OF MEDICINES

by Ogden Tanner

AND THE EDITORS OF TIME-LIFE BOOKS

LIBRARY OF HEALTH / TIME-LIFE BOOKS / ALEXANDRIA, VIRGINIA

THE AUTHOR:
Ogden Tanner, formerly an editor on the staff of Time-Life Books, has written volumes for several Time-Life Books series, including Human Behavior, The TIME-LIFE Encyclopedia of Gardening and The American Wilderness. Trained in architecture at Princeton University, he served as an editor of *House and Home* and *Architectural Forum.* Mr. Tanner was born in New York and now lives in Connecticut.

THE CONSULTANTS:
Dr. James W. Long is Director of Health Services for the National Science Foundation, consultant to the Food and Drug Administration and Assistant Clinical Professor, Department of Medicine at the George Washington University School of Medicine in Washington, D.C. He served as a delegate to the U.S. Pharmacopeial Convention and directed the Drug Information Association. He is the author of *The Essential Guide to Prescription Drugs.*

Donald O. Fedder is Assistant Professor of Pharmacy Practice and Administrative Sciences and Director of Community Pharmacy and Professional Experience Programs at the University of Maryland School of Pharmacy in Baltimore. Mr. Fedder served on the American Pharmaceutical Association's Advisory Committee on Drug Interactions and is Vice Chairman of the Maryland High Blood Pressure Coordinating Council.

For information about any Time-Life book, please write:
Reader Information, Time-Life Books,
541 North Fairbanks Court, Chicago, Illinois 60611.

First printing.
Published simultaneously in Canada.
School and library distribution by Silver Burdett Company, Morristown, New Jersey.

TIME-LIFE is a trademark of Time Incorporated U.S.A.

Library of Congress Cataloguing in Publication Data
The Editors of Time-Life Books
  The Prudent Use of Medicines
  (Library of Health)
  Bibliography p.
  Includes index.
  1. Drugs—Popular works.
  I. Time-Life Books.   II. Series.
RM301.15.P78   615'.1   81-9273
ISBN 0-8094-3772-4   AACR2
ISBN 0-8094-3771-6 (lib. bdg.)
ISBN 0-8094-3370-8 (retail ed.)

LIBRARY OF HEALTH

Editor: Martin Mann
Editorial Staff for *The Prudent Use of Medicines*
Senior Editor: William Frankel
Assistant Editor: Phyllis K. Wise
Designer: Albert Sherman
Picture Editor: Jane N. Coughran
Text Editors: Laura Longley, C. Tyler Mathisen, Paul N. Mathless
Writers: Deborah Berger-Turnbull, Peter Kaufman, Brian McGinn
Researchers: Megan Helene Barnett (principal), Judy French, Carlos Vidal Greth, Jonn Ethan Hankins, Melva Morgan Holloman, Norma E. Kennedy, Sara Mark, Fran Moshos, Trudy W. Pearson, Jules Taylor
Assistant Designer: Cynthia T. Richardson
Copy Coordinators: Margery duMond, Stephen G. Hyslop, Diane Ullius Jarrett
Picture Coordinator: Rebecca Christoffersen
Editorial Assistant: Nana Heinbaugh Juarbe
Special Contributors: Stanley Cloud, Christopher S. Conner, Susan Perry Dawson, Norman Kolpas, Patricia Molino, Frederick King Poole, Lydia Preston (writers); Barbara Lerner, David F. Long (researchers)

EDITORIAL OPERATIONS
Production Director: Feliciano Madrid
Assistants: Peter A. Inchauteguiz, Karen A. Meyerson
Copy Processing: Gordon E. Buck
Quality Control Director: Robert L. Young
Assistant: James J. Cox
Associates: Daniel J. McSweeney, Michael G. Wight
Art Coordinator: Anne B. Landry
Copy Room Director: Susan B. Galloway
Assistants: Celia Beattie, Ricki Tarlow

Correspondents: Elisabeth Kraemer, Helga Kohl (Bonn); Margot Hapgood, Dorothy Bacon, Lesley Coleman (London); Susan Jonas, Lucy T. Voulgaris (New York); Maria Vincenza Aloisi, Josephine du Brusle (Paris); Ann Natanson (Rome). Valuable assistance was also given by: Wibo Van De Linde (Amsterdam); Nat Harrison (Cairo); Robert Kroon (Geneva); Bing Wong (Hong Kong); Judy Aspinall, Jeremy Lawrence, Pippa Pridham (London); John Dunn (Melbourne); Felix Rosenthal (Moscow); William Campbell, Alistair Matheson (Nairobi); Marcia Gauger (New Delhi); Carolyn T. Chubet, Diane Cook, Miriam Hsia, Christina Lieberman, Alexandra Mezey (New York); Leonora Dodsworth, Mimi Murphy (Rome); Janet Zich (San Francisco); Edwin Reingold (Tokyo); Traudl Lessing (Vienna).

CONTENTS

CHAPTER 1

A pill for every ill?

Potent remedies of the ancients
Modern miracles in molds
Every drug a poison
The tranquilizer boom
Fake pills, real cures
Weighing special risks
How to get the most from any medicine

"A desire to take medicines," wrote the Canadian physician Sir William Osler in 1891, "is, perhaps, the great feature which distinguishes man from other animals." If Osler's wry observation was true in his time, it is even more strikingly true today. People take medicines, and take them, and take them—in staggering amounts.

By the 1980s, Americans were consuming yearly more than six billion dollars' worth of nonprescription cough and cold remedies, painkillers, vitamins and health tonics, antacids, laxatives and a host of other products, ranging from eyewashes to wart-removers. On any given day about 40 million Americans—almost one fifth of the population—used one nonprescription remedy or another. In addition, two thirds of the population had used prescription drugs at some time, and about 75 million had taken them regularly. These drugs, available only by prescription and dispensed by a licensed pharmacist, are too potent and too hazardous to use without precise instructions from a doctor—yet they, too, are obviously taken in awe-inspiring quantities.

Steering a safe course through this ocean of medication calls for caution and common sense, informed by expert guidance from physicians and pharmacists. The caution and common sense must be exercised by every adult when taking any drugs for any ill, serious or minor. In turning to nonprescription drugs for minor problems, the patient is his own doctor—he diagnoses his ailments and prescribes for himself the medicines he hopes will cure them. To do so wisely, he needs reliable data so that he can decide first that the ailment does not require a physician's attention, second that it should be treated with some medicine rather than being left alone to take care of itself, and finally, which drug should be used—not all of them are effective, even for the light-duty work they are meant to accomplish.

Prescription drugs are inherently dangerous—not only are most of them much more potent than those sold over the counter but they are generally more complex. Indeed, regulations issued by the Food and Drug Administration (FDA) in 1945 forbid prescription labels that give instructions for choosing and using drugs; it was felt that such instructions would encourage dangerous self-treatment. Yet even though physicians are responsible for prescribing drugs, they need the active participation of an informed patient. The prudent user of prescription medicines must know what kind of information to give the doctor, what kind to get from him, how to follow his instructions—and how to tell whether the prescription is working the way it is supposed to.

The pharmacist who fills prescriptions and sells nonprescription remedies is perhaps the most accessible—and inexpensive—dispenser of expert advice on effective and safe use of medicines. For over-the-counter drugs he is the one health professional readily available to guide an individual in handling his own health problem. For both prescription and nonprescription drugs, the pharmacist often has the broadest, most up-to-date information on drug effects, including recently discovered side effects and interactions between drugs and other substances. He also can point to economies in drug

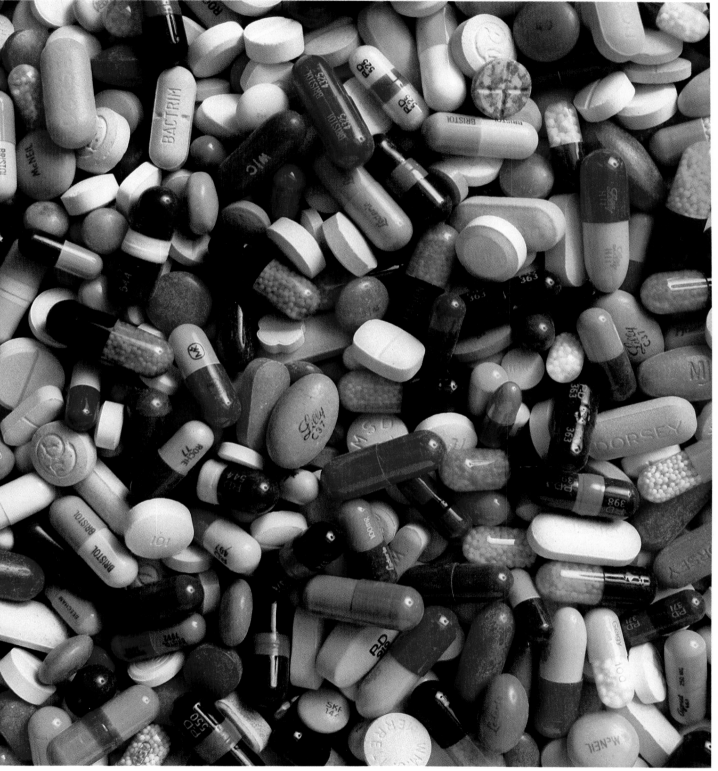

Looking like candies in a confectioner's bin, this jumble of some 100 tablets and capsules is a tiny sample of more than a quarter million drug products sold to treat ailments ranging from cancer to the common cold. American pharmacists fill close to 1.4 billion doctors' prescriptions each year, and annual sales of nonprescription remedies exceed five billion dollars.

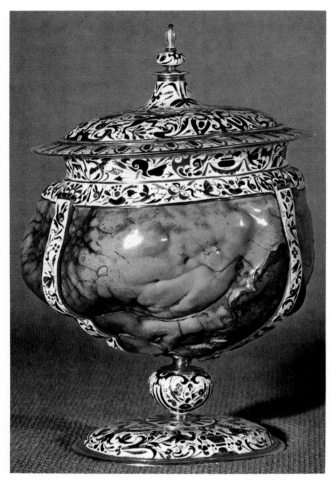

This 16th Century European bowl is carved from dappled amber bezoar stone—a hardened inorganic mass extracted from the stomach or gall bladder of a wild goat or gazelle—and is set within an enameled gold frame. In Europe and the Near East from the 12th to the mid-18th Centuries, pulverized bezoar stone was particularly prized as a poison antidote.

purchases by explaining when and when not to save money by buying in quantity or by selecting drugs by their chemical content—indicated by "generic" names—rather than by brand. Armed with such information, the prudent user of medicines is in a position to control a large part of his own health care and to participate intelligently with his physician and pharmacist in obtaining safe and effective drug therapy at reasonable cost.

A practical understanding of drugs used is more important now than it has ever been. Although medicines go further back in human history than the written evidence records, never have there been so many with such powerful effects. Moreover, the scientific research that has preceded (or, often, followed) the discovery of new medicines has revealed much about the mechanisms of drug action, and this knowledge is one of the keys to prudent use. It is far from complete—the methods of action of about 40 per cent of some of the most commonly used drugs are still only guessed at—but the information that has been gained is invaluable in deciding when and how to use what.

Potent remedies of the ancients

The understanding of drugs is new despite their long history. Many remedies in use for centuries—some for millennia—were potent and effective: opium as a painkiller, foxglove extract (digitalis) as a heart stimulant, aspirin-like willow-bark concoctions as a fever cure, cinchona bark (quinine) as a malaria treatment. Many more were fearsome enough to have shocked the patient out of his illness. Robert Boyle, the 17th Century British "father of modern chemistry," who first defined chemical elements, advised eating soap to cure patients with bloody urine and drinking mercury in beer to get rid of intestinal worms.

Whether their prescriptions were sage or foolish, medicine men of the past never knew how they worked. Lacking fundamental knowledge of the body's physical and chemical processes, they could only look for substances in nature and apply them by guess and instinct. The first rational advances in medicine in the 18th Century were the result of observed effects rather than discovered causes: Vaccination, for example, protected people against infection by the smallpox virus 100 years before anyone knew viruses existed; scurvy was cured by citrus fruits at least 175 years before the active ingredient, vitamin C, was identified.

The 19th Century saw the major advances in the development of medicines. First, chemists learned how to isolate active medicinal ingredients from the plant tissues in which they were hidden. The extraction of morphine from raw opium, quinine from cinchona bark, atropine from belladonna, and other potent drugs from natural materials meant that man no longer had to take the imperfect offerings of nature as they came, but could refine them to their purest and most potent form. He was now able, furthermore, to improve on nature by cooking up synthetic compounds that were similar to natural chemicals but superior to them. Aspirin—acetylsalicylic acid—is a synthetic not found in willow bark, and it lowers fevers and eases headaches far better than any of the related chemicals extracted from willow bark.

Effective medicines multiplied in the 20th Century as researchers applied their growing laboratory skills to a deepening knowledge of bacteria—and, later, viruses—to gain the upper hand over deadly infectious diseases. Vaccines have now wiped smallpox from the face of the earth; it is a disease that no longer exists. Diphtheria, which killed an average of 1,830 people a year in England and Wales between 1940 and 1944, caused no deaths in 1969. In 1933 nearly 800 Americans died of polio; in 1978 only 13 died of that illness. Syphilis not only killed at a rate of 17.3 per 100,000 in 1925 but also caused psychosis; by 1978 the syphilis death rate was one in a million.

More recently, tranquilizers have brought some severe mental diseases under control and have enabled many once-hopeless patients to leave the care of mental hospitals. Other drugs have allowed millions of diabetics, heart patients and sufferers from high blood pressure to lead normal lives. Still other medicines have improved the plight of victims of such rarer ills as hemophilia and Parkinson's disease.

Even dreaded cancer is being put under control by chemical treatment in combination with surgery and X-rays. The cure rate for breast cancer went from 50 per cent to nearly 70 per cent in about 30 years, for cancer of the womb from 61 to 81 per cent. For Hodgkins disease, a cancer of the body's infection-fighting system, a combination of four powerful chemicals brought the cure rate to over 50 per cent.

The drugs that have won so many battles—and even several wars—against disease and death have come rapidly. While the modern era of chemotherapy began with the clinical use of sulfanilamide in 1936, most of these "miracle drugs" have been discovered or created since World War II, in what has been called a golden age of drug development. Antibiotics—especially penicillin—opened the golden age in the 1940s. The 1950s saw the introduction of the first modern mind-altering drugs—both the powerful chemicals for severe mental disorders and the so-called minor tranquilizers, the first of a growing family of widely used drugs that deal with anxiety and stress. In this decade also came the first blood-thinners (anticoagulants) for heart attack and stroke victims, the first diuretics for controlling high blood pressure by eliminating body fluids, and the first modifier of the body's own control systems for pregnancy (the Pill).

Modern miracles in molds

It sometimes happens that the history of a single drug or class of drugs recapitulates the long, slow evolution from hit-or-miss remedies to the sophisticated manipulation of molecules. So it was with the family of bacteria-killers called antibiotics and their most famous member, penicillin. The story is familiar in part: During World War II, a substance derived from a mold was found to cure bacterial infection in the body. But the full story has its roots in the distant past and is continuing even today.

To begin with, there was nothing new about using molds or earth to fight germs. The Chinese did it more than 2,500 years ago, by applying moldy soybean curd to such skin infections as boils and carbuncles. Mud was used by the ancient Egyptians to treat sores. Over the millennia, similar substances were tried, with mixed and meaningless results—some may have cured, others almost certainly killed, and still others had no effect whatever. Only with the modern understanding of microorganisms that live in soil and water

BASIL
Old herbals recommend basil tea for
stomach and intestinal ailments, such
as cramps, constipation and vomiting. It is
also said to relieve headaches and,
when honey is added, coughs.

DILL
The seeds of dill, like those of many
fragrant plants, can be chewed to cure
bad breath. They can also be brewed in a
tea said to be useful in relieving
stomach-aches, flatulence and insomnia.

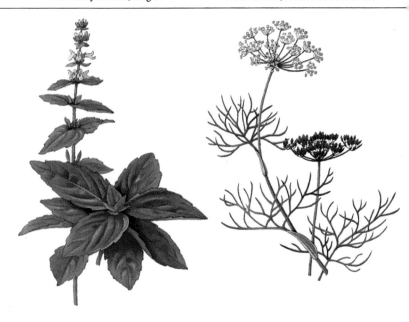

Potions from the herb garden

Many of the herbs commonly used in patent and traditional
medicines can be grown at home, in outdoor herb gardens or
indoors on a sunny window sill. Some of the most popular of
these plants appear at right and below. A few work: Balm
made from aloe *(top, third from left),* a traditional remedy for
burns and sores, contains anthraquinones, which are known
to be effective soothing agents. However, the curative powers of many herbal remedies are now believed to depend
more on the way they are used than on intrinsic pharmacologic action. Herbs are usually brewed into teas, which may
help relax constricted breathing passages, quiet a nagging
cough or calm the digestive system; but it is the hot water
or vapor, not the herb, that does the job. Similarly, herb-
flavored warm milk does help induce sleep because milk
contains tryptophan, a mild relaxant.

One of the most widely used herbal remedies, garlic, employed in many forms as a cure for many ills, has no therapeutic effect that can be detected. Yet even the most skeptical
scientists are reluctant to scoff. Snakeroot powder was sold
in India for 3,000 years to relieve "mental agitation." Not
until the 1950s was it recognized as a source of reserpine, a
potent tranquilizer and blood-pressure medicine.

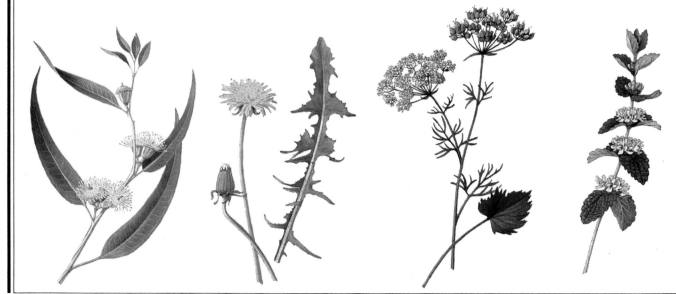

EUCALYPTUS
Mature leaves of the eucalyptus tree,
which are sold in many health-food
stores, can be boiled in water to generate
vapors that are claimed to relieve
asthma and other respiratory ailments.

DANDELION
A tea brewed from dandelion, using one or
all parts of the plant, is effective as a
mild laxative. Its supposed value in
relieving stiff joints and rheumatism,
however, is questionable.

ANISE
A tea made from the seeds of the anise
plant is another folk remedy for
indigestion and stomach-aches. The
crushed seeds are often used to flavor
warm milk for a helpful sleeping potion.

HOREHOUND
Many old-fashioned herbals prescribe hot
horehound tea to relieve coughs and
congestion of the lungs. In addition the
tea, when it is taken cold, is said to
serve as a good stomach tonic.

ALOE
The long, fleshy leaves of this common houseplant are filled with a gelatinous juice that, applied to the skin, effectively relieves the discomfort of sunburn, insect bites and minor cuts and scratches.

CHICORY
A tea brewed from the root or leaves of chicory is said to improve appetite and digestion. Its flowers and leaves, when boiled and wrapped in a compress, purportedly soothe inflammation.

GREAT MULLEIN
Mullein tea, made with the plant's leaves and flowers, is recommended by herbalists as a remedy for coughs, hoarseness and sore throats. Vapors from the tea may help ease breathing.

PARSLEY
Chewing fresh parsley is an old folk remedy for bad breath. A tea made from the plant's seeds and leaves is said to relieve coughs and, when rubbed into the scalp, to kill lice.

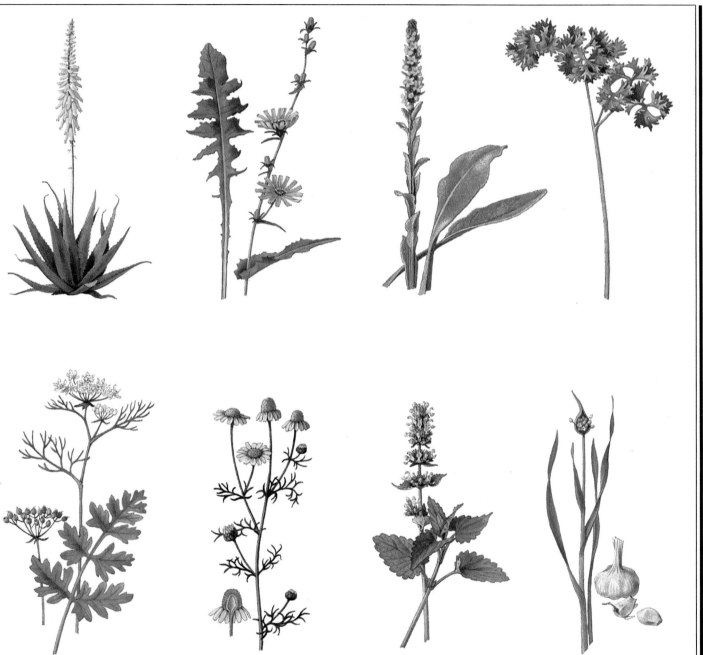

CORIANDER
Tea made from coriander seeds is believed to improve the appetite and to relieve stomach-aches. Vapors from coriander tea are also used in the treatment of sinus and respiratory problems.

GERMAN CAMOMILE
Drinking camomile-flower tea, an unproven remedy for nervous tension and insomnia, may prompt an allergic reaction—especially in people with known allergies to pollen.

CATNIP
Catnip tea is widely believed to reduce fevers, relieve headaches and calm nerves. An infusion, with two or three tablespoonfuls taken several times daily, is prescribed for flatulence.

GARLIC
A popular cure-all in herbal folklore, garlic is believed to be especially effective in relieving digestive problems. Some herbalists claim it lowers blood pressure and prevents cancer.

did the development of medicines drawn from microorganisms begin to gather momentum.

In the 1870s no fewer than three investigators, including the great English surgeon Joseph Lister, independently noted that a fungus of the genus Penicillium had the power to inhibit the growth of bacteria in its vicinity. Some 20 years later, in 1896, an obscure French medical student named Ernest Duchesne made the discovery all over again.

By the 1930s, a hunt for the active ingredients responsible for these effects was going on in many parts of the world. In 1939, at the Rockefeller Institute for Medical Research, the French-born American microbiologist René Dubos isolated tyrothricin, the first antibiotic to be used in clinical trials; two years later he isolated gramicidin, its active component. At Rutgers University, in New Jersey, another microbiologist, Selman Waksman, started a search in 1939 for a tuberculosis remedy in soil-dwelling bacteria. Five years and 10,000 soil samples later, he came up with streptomycin. And at Oxford University, in 1938, the English scientists Howard Florey and Ernst Chain began what they called ''a systematic investigation of the chemical and biological properties of the antibacterial substances produced by bacteria and moulds.''

One of the first objects of their research was a curiosity reported in the medical literature: the well-known action of Penicillium fungus. In 1928, while studying staphylococcus bacteria in London, the bacteriologist Alexander Fleming had noticed that the surface of one bacterial culture had been contaminated by Penicillium, and that some of the germs were dying. Another researcher might have simply discarded the culture. Instead, Fleming set out to study the powerful fungus and to test its action against other bacteria. He found that penicillin, a substance secreted by Penicillium, killed some types of bacteria while leaving others untouched, and that it was harmless to laboratory animals and to the white cells of human blood.

There, for all practical purposes, his investigation ended. As a bacteriologist, he was intrigued by penicillin's selective action, and suggested that it might be used in the laboratory to isolate types of bacteria in mixed cultures. He tried it out as an antiseptic salve, with good but not striking success. But he never thought of introducing it into the bloodstream, where its antibacterial power could take effect, and he found that penicillin was not only difficult to grow but very unstable. More than a decade after making his discovery, Fleming confessed that, at the time, penicillin hardly seemed worth the trouble of producing it.

In 1940, Florey and Chain took the next crucial step. They partly purified penicillin and tested it, by injection, against infections in laboratory mice, then in human beings. The results, Florey later wrote, were ''so gratifying as to be at times almost unbelievable.'' Physicians had never before had an effective method of treating, rather than preventing, a wide range of bacterial infections. Now, such scourges as pneumonia and meningitis could be cured with apparently miraculous ease, and the wounds of battle—so grievously plentiful in the world of the 1940s—could be made safe from infection.

At this point modern pharmaceutical technology turned hope into reality. Like Fleming before them, Florey and Chain were able to make penicillin only in pitifully small quantities: During their clinical trials they were forced at times to retrieve used penicillin from the body wastes of their patients. But after moving to the safety of the United States, and working with scientists at a U.S. Department of Agriculture laboratory in Peoria, Illinois, they solved the problem of large-scale production.

Improved mediums for growing Penicillium, more productive strains of the fungus itself and a technique for breeding the fungus by deep cultures in vat fermenters rather than by surface cultures in bottles—such advances made penicillin available in plenty. By 1943 the Americans who had contributed to the new methods of manufacture had put the drug into commercial production; by the end of the War, there was enough for soldier and civilian alike. In modern pharmaceutical factories, the yields achieved by Chain and Florey in the 1940s are multiplied thousands of times.

To counter the kinds of bacteria that the original strain of penicillin did not kill, scientists scoured the world for new antibiotics. They tested molds, fungi and soil samples by the hundreds of thousands, and came up with whole families of potent drugs—including Selman Waksman's streptomycin, the first medicine effective against tuberculosis; erythromycin, which is effective against such diseases as diphtheria and whooping cough; the tetracyclines, effective against such diseases as Rocky Mountain spotted fever, typhoid fever and gonorrhea. And penicillin developed into a family of 23 different drugs, used clinically or under active investigation, each with its own range of potency and its own special applications.

Eventually, however, this run of success began to suffer setbacks. Not only were some bacteria naturally resistant to penicillin, but bacteria that had once been vulnerable to it began to develop resistance. These newly resistant bacterial strains were mutants—genetic variations that survived because they had evolved structures that penicillin could not attack, or had come to produce secretions that attacked penicillin itself. In the 1950s, for example, penicillin was used to cure gonorrhea; by the 1980s, it failed 20 per cent of the time against certain strains. Some doctors began to think of the traditional antibiotics as "one-shot" remedies—if the drugs did not effect a cure on the first try, rapidly developing mutant bacteria could render them ineffective thereafter.

Once again, as it had back in the 1940s, a solution began to emerge from the laboratory—but this time at a much higher level of sophistication. For one thing, scientists had cracked the riddle of penicillin's structure. All the diverse forms of the drug, whatever the differences in their molecules, have one feature in common: a so-called beta-lactam ring, consisting of a tight core of four atoms, three carbon and one nitrogen. Linked to the beta-lactam ring is a second ring of five atoms, the thiazolidine ring; and from the two rings radiate variable chains of atoms—carbon, nitrogen, oxygen and hydrogen. By synthesizing new chains and linking them to the central ring, researchers can create new penicillins to fight resistant bacterial mutations.

Penicillin is not the only beta-lactam antibiotic. The cephalosporins also have the characteristic central ring. In the cephalosporins, however, the beta-lactam ring is linked to a second ring of six atoms rather than five. Literally thousands of penicillins and cephalosporins have been produced

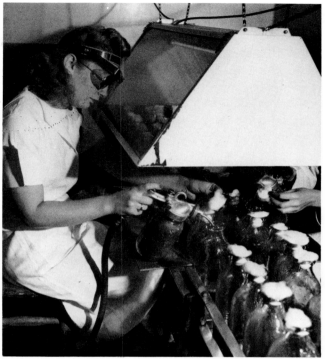

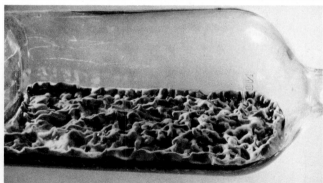

In a photograph taken shortly after penicillin came into use, a technician injects spores into jars to grow penicillin-bearing fungus on the surface of the liquid (bottom)—a method giving meager yields. By 1943 a way was found to grow the fungus throughout the medium instead of just on top—vastly increasing supplies in time to save countless lives in World War II.

in the laboratory; even more are still to come. Most are ineffective—but as researchers gain knowledge of the intricate beta-lactam structures, new antibiotics emerge, tailormade to meet new bacterial challenges. By the beginning of the 1980s, these researchers were working on a third generation of cephalosporins, typified by such drugs as moxalactam *(page 82)*; these new drugs had a wider spectrum of activity and stronger weapons against bacterial resistance than any known before.

Rejiggering molecules to make new medicines is one of two revolutionary techniques that promise a new golden age of drug development. The other is genetic engineering—so-called recombinant DNA technology—which can actually create new forms of life by taking unimaginably small snippets of heredity-controlling DNA from one organism and splicing them into the DNA of another. This gene-splicing creates a new type of organism that can be put to work manufacturing drugs.

About one fifth of present-day medicines—such as antibiotics—are products of chemical activity in living organisms. Gene-splicing can isolate the key DNA components of these medicine-making organisms and transplant them into abundant, easily controlled bacteria and fungi. These organisms thus are genetically programed to act as microscopic pharmaceutical factories for producing unlimited quantities of substances now available only in minute amounts or in impure, hazardous forms.

Already this revolutionary technique has led to the creation of a synthetic hormone—identical to the one produced naturally by the human body—that helps control substances involved in growth and in diabetes. In addition, human insulin, the body chemical that is lacking in many diabetics and must be supplied by injection to keep them alive, has also been produced by such alteration of the common bacterium *Escherichia coli*. Because this synthetic is indistinguishable from the body's own insulin, it is more effective in treating diabetes than the animal insulin commonly used; it is also cheaper—a tank containing about 500 gallons of *E. coli* broth yields more than three ounces of purified insulin, as much as could be produced from nearly a ton of animal

glands. Even more promising is the use of gene-spliced *E. coli* to make interferon, a substance that may help prevent virus diseases and stop cancers.

Every drug a poison

Yet even the most miraculous miracle drug harbors within it powerful danger. Most medicines, whether synthesized in a test tube or extracted from natural substances, are chemicals that are foreign to the body and can be poisonous to one degree or another. Even those that are compounds normally present in the body, such as insulin, can cause harm. There simply is no such thing as a perfectly safe drug. Even familiar, seemingly unthreatening medicines such as aspirin and antihistamines can have multiple effects that range from mild discomfort to lethal shock.

Each drug's potential for ill, weighed against the good sought from it—the so-called risk-benefit ratio—provides a gauge useful in deciding whether to take a drug. Aspirin, for example, usually presents only modest risks, and the benefits often sought from it, such as relief from a headache, seem similarly modest. When the risk increases, as it does if the presence of stomach ulcers brings hazard of internal bleeding from the irritation of aspirin's acid, the serious risk may outweigh the benefit; it may be wiser to endure the headache or use another agent such as acetaminophen. A cancer patient, on the other hand, may be justified in trying extremely toxic medicines because they hold the only remaining promise of arresting the disease and prolonging his life.

Circumstances may weigh against the use of otherwise acceptable drugs: A farmer, for example, should pause before using an antibiotic that may also cause sensitivity to sunlight. Women, who are normally free to take any drug a man can take, should be extremely wary of any drug when they are pregnant, for many medicines can affect unborn babies and some affect them disastrously.

Such problems are complicated by the abundance of drugs available; for some disorders there are as many as 40 or 50 different medicines and it is sometimes difficult for doctors or patients to decide which one to use. The growing array of effective medicines has also led many people to believe that

Homeopathy: fighting fire with fire

Thousands of patients disillusioned by modern medical practice find unconventional relief in homeopathy, a system of treatment employing as remedies a variety of natural substances that can cause the same symptoms as the ailment—in effect, fighting fire with fire. Founded at the beginning of the 19th Century by the German physician and linguist Dr. Samuel Hahnemann, homeopathy originally provided a humane alternative to the brutal bleedings, purgings and enemas of 19th Century European medicine.

Hahnemann gained wide popularity in Europe after employing his methods to treat successfully 179 victims of a killer typhoid epidemic in 1813. German and Swiss immigrants brought Hahnemann's techniques to the United States with them in the 1820s; by the beginning of the 20th Century there were 22 homeopathic medical schools, more than 100 hospitals and 10,000 homeopathic doctors in the United States alone. Today there probably are fewer than 1,000 American physicians, including Ohio's Dr. Maesimund B. Panos (overleaf), who continue to practice homeopathy, although in recent years there has been increasing interest in the Hahnemann approach.

The obscurity of Hahnemann's Laws of Homeopathy—and the lack of supporting scientific evidence for them—undoubtedly contributed to the decline in the popularity of homeopathic medicine. The cardinal principle, known as the Law of Similars, holds that a substance capable of producing symptoms of a particular disease in a healthy person also is capable of alleviating those symptoms and curing the disease in an ill person. A companion tenet, the Law of Potentization, states that the potency of a curative agent increases as the substance is diluted—a paradox that permits the safe use of toxic materials.

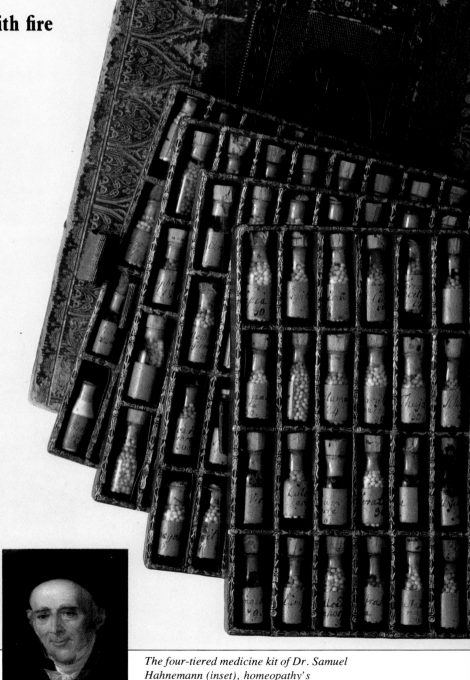

The four-tiered medicine kit of Dr. Samuel Hahnemann (inset), homeopathy's founder, held some 200 medicine vials. The modern homeopathic pharmacopeia has about 2,000 remedies, made from vegetable, mineral and animal substances.

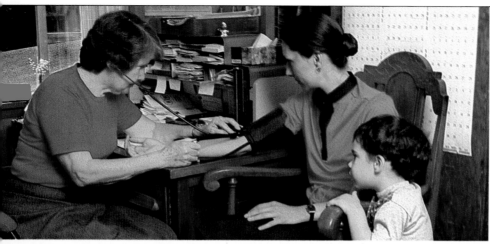

Combining orthodox medical technique with homeopathy, Dr. Maesimund Panos takes a patient's blood pressure in her Tipp City, Ohio, office. Like most homeopaths, Dr. Panos is an M.D., with a degree in family medicine from Ohio State University.

After matching her patient's symptoms against patterns recorded in homeopathic literature, Dr. Panos selects a single remedy from a roster of drugs that can cause similar indications. Her office stock includes more than 500 medicines.

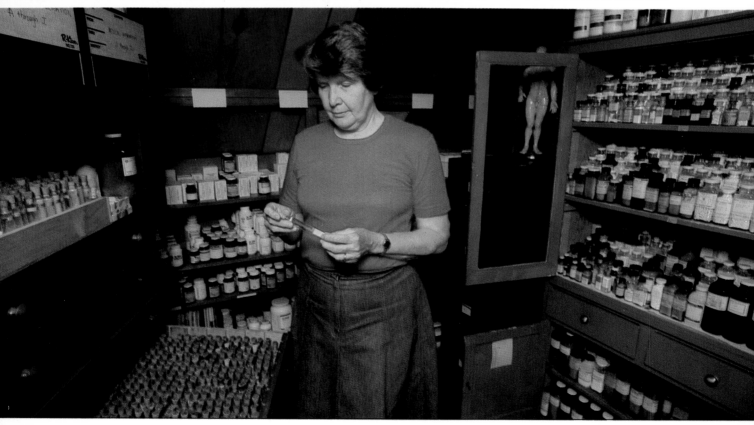

The 15 homeopathic remedies listed below are included in a 28-item home-remedy kit designed by Dr. Panos for her patients, some of whom live as far as 1,300 miles from her office. The source of each medicine is indicated in parentheses after the technical name. The remedies are intended for self-treatment of the minor injuries and ailments listed in the right-hand column.

MEDICINE:	PRESCRIBED FOR:
Allium cepa (red onion)	Colds involving sneezing, watery eyes and nose, and laryngitis
Antimonium tartaricum (tartar emetic)	Bronchitis accompanied by wheezing cough, cold sweat and pallor
Apis mellifica (honeybee)	Insect bites such as mosquito bites, involving swelling, itching and redness
Arsenicum album (arsenic)	Upset stomach (indigestion), accompanied by vomiting or diarrhea
Cantharis (Spanish fly)	Cystitis involving painful urination; also pain of burns and scalds
Carbo vegetabilis (vegetable charcoal)	Exhaustion; weakness after illness; also upset stomach accompanied by heartburn or gas
Gelsemium sempervirens (yellow jasmine)	Influenza; sore throat with reddened tonsils; also head colds or tension headaches
Ignatia amara (St.-Ignatius's-bean)	Prolonged emotional upset accompanied by depression or insomnia
Ledum palustre (marsh tea)	Puncture wounds, stings, bites, eye injuries or sprained ankle
Magnesia phosphorica (phosphate of magnesia)	Spasmodic pain such as leg cramps, menstrual cramps or colic
Mercurius vivus (mercury)	Tonsillitis, abscessed ears, boils or gum disease, accompanied by profuse sweating, weakness and trembling
Nux vomica (poison nut)	Hangover; also ill effects of spicy foods or overeating
Ruta graveolens (rue)	Shinbone injury; also strains, particularly of the tendons
Spongia tosta (roasted sponge)	Croup or dry cough beginning in the throat, accompanied by a feeling of suffocation
Sulphur (sulfur)	Chronic skin diseases involving dry, itchy skin, with a burning sensation

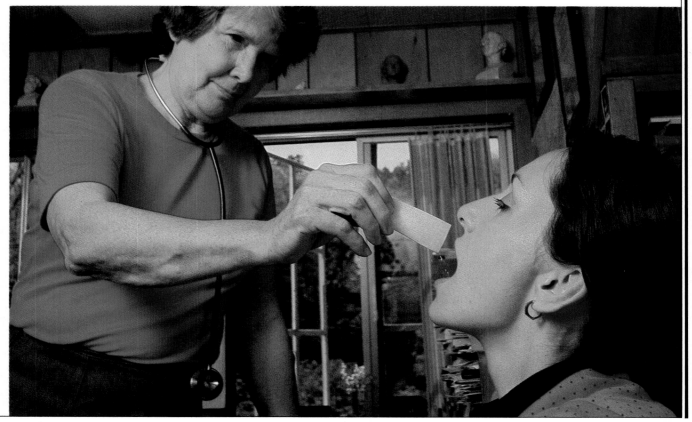

Dr. Panos administers a single dose of the prescribed remedy—Agave, made from the century plant and used to treat skin ailments—to her patient. Practitioners of classical homeopathy administer only one medicine at a time.

there must be a remedy for everything, even the slightest discomfort—"a pill for every ill." This notion has promoted a sometimes indiscriminate consumption of medicines. Anyone can be harmed if drugs are taken too often or in amounts greater than recommended, or if they are consumed with certain other drugs or foods that cause unpleasant or dangerous interactions *(pages 88-89)*.

Blame for an "overmedicated society" has been laid at almost every door. Scarcely a week passes without some furor over drug misuse. A rock star mixes too many pills and takes dramatic, terminal leave of his fans. The acting chairwoman of a Congressional committee declares that a doctor often tells a male patient to work out his problem in the gym, while a female with the same symptoms is likely to be given a prescription for Valium.

The tranquilizer boom

The ubiquitous minor tranquilizers are perhaps the most controversial of the modern miracle drugs. The first, meprobamate, was introduced in 1955 under the trade name Miltown and it was soon followed by chlordiazepoxide (Librium), diazepam (Valium) and several others. These drugs can be both effective and safe for occasional, short-term use in relieving worries and tensions, especially during critical periods of stress, and in treating conditions such as alcohol withdrawal, painful muscle spasms and certain types of epilepsy. Unfortunately, their use is not limited to those purposes. They can prove addictive, and they can interact lethally with other drugs that depress nerve activity, such as alcohol and barbiturates.

The indiscriminate use of some of these tranquilizers eventually became so widespread that the trade name Valium entered common usage. In one Hollywood movie, the leading character suffers an acute anxiety attack in a busy department store. As he gasps for breath before a small crowd of onlooking shoppers, a companion turns and asks if anyone has a Valium. Every person in the crowd instantly reaches into pocket or handbag and proffers a bottle of the pills.

This bit of comic fiction may not be far off the mark: According to Jere Goyan, former Commissioner of the FDA,

an average of one out of every three Americans receives a prescription for a tranquilizer every year.

The notoriety accorded the overuse of tranquilizers and other relaxants had a striking result. Doctors began to prescribe them, and patients to use them, less and less. The National Prescription Audit, a private survey, found that prescriptions for the benzodiazepines, a group of minor tranquilizers, dropped from a peak of more than 88 million in 1975 to some 62 million in 1979. During the same period prescriptions for sleeping pills also dropped, from 46 million to 32.5 million, and for painkillers from 120 million to 104 million a year.

A growing sense that drugs were being overused, in fact, led to a slight decline in all prescribing in the late 1970s. Dr. Richard A. Crout, director of the FDA's Bureau of Drugs, attributed the drop to adverse publicity, to educational campaigns aimed at both physicians and patients, and to a growing popularity of jogging, yoga exercises and other alternate solutions to everyday stress. Said Dr. Robert L. DuPont, former head of the National Institute on Drug Abuse, "Some patients these days look at you with distrust if you even mention drugs."

Whether this decline indicates a real change in drug use is unclear; in the 1980s the number of prescriptions began to increase slightly. The human urge to take medicines remains strong, and some doctors write prescriptions simply because some patients demand it; they may be disappointed or even angry if they leave the doctor's office without a little piece of paper bearing some impressive, if incomprehensible, markings—a sort of written guarantee that they need only take this medicine and they will be well again.

Fake pills, real cures

Physicians accede to the demand for medicines for a very good reason. They know that anything they do, if done with authority and confidence, may help make the patient well. A relatively safe concoction, even though it has no direct action on the biological systems of the body, may not only satisfy the patient but may actually bring about a cure—through the mysterious, somewhat magical process known as the placebo effect (after the Latin word meaning "I shall please"). This phenomenon is responsible for much success in treating minor ailments—and a surprising number of major ones, up to and including the pain of cancer. It depends not on the actual chemical make-up of the medicine but on the patient's own attitude: his faith in the doctor, his expectations about some new cure or simply his determination to rise above the problem and get well.

Dozens of studies have shown that about one third of all sufferers from a wide variety of illnesses derived pain relief from placebos, usually innocuous sugar pills carefully prepared to look and taste like bona fide medicines and administered as if they were. Placebos relieve not only simple headaches but even severe pain following major surgery. In one investigation an injection of a placebo, rather than morphine, was found to help 42 per cent of postoperative patients. In treating anxiety, placebos have proved still more effective in some cases, helping more than half of the subjects in some experiments.

Placebo power can work in reverse, too: After being warned about the side effects—dizziness, headache and stomach upset—associated with certain drugs, an appreciable number of people given placebos masquerading as the culprit drugs experienced those very effects. Commented the world-famed medical missionary Albert Schweitzer: "The witch doctor succeeds for the same reason all the rest of us succeed. Each patient carries his own doctor inside him. They come to us not knowing that truth. We are at our best when we give the doctor who resides within each patient a chance to go to work."

One of the most intriguing, and convincing, examples of the placebo effect is the experience of Norman Cousins, the writer and magazine editor, as told in his book *Anatomy of an Illness*. After a trip to Russia, Cousins came down with a rare and painful disease affecting the collagen, the body's connective tissue; one specialist said his chances of recovering were 1 in 500. Cousins was unwilling to accept that verdict. With the encouragement of his doctor, he decided to stop taking a battery of harsh drugs and instead try a different course of therapy: humor, in the form of old Marx Brothers movies and television programs shown on a screen he had set up in his hospital room, plus massive intravenous doses of vitamin C. Cousins had read that people suffering from collagen disease have a vitamin C deficiency, and insisted on taking it, although scientific studies had cast doubt on its use as a treatment for collagen disease.

His self-treatment worked. Gradually, the pain subsided enough for Cousins to sleep. At first so weak that he could barely move his limbs, he slowly regained enough strength and mobility to go back to his magazine job. Cousins was convinced that three things helped him get well—the strong support of his doctor, laughter and vitamin C. Of his massive intake of a supposedly irrelevant vitamin he said, "It is quite possible that this treatment—like everything else I did—was a demonstration of the placebo effect."

How placebos actually work is not known, but some researchers believe the pain-relieving effect may result from the release of chemicals in the brain called endorphins, often referred to as natural morphines. "Studies show," Cousins observed, "that up to 90 per cent of patients who reach out for medical help are suffering from self-limiting disorders well within the range of the body's own healing powers. The placebo is not so much a pill as a process. The process begins with the patient's confidence in the doctor and extends through to the full functioning of his own immunological and healing system."

Whatever the precise mechanism may turn out to be, the placebo process is an indisputable medical phenomenon—so real and powerful, in fact, that it can throw off the results of drug testing in humans and must routinely be allowed for through the so-called double-blind test *(Chapter 6)*.

Ancient medicines depended largely on the placebo effect. When they worked it was because patients believed they would work. Even the mud used by the early Egyptians to treat sores could rarely have contained enough antibiotic chemicals to kill bacterial infections. Once in a while it may have. Such occasional successes presumably established its reputation, and a reputation for success is enough; subsequent cures can be gained purely from the placebo effect.

Modern medicines are different. Those approved for sale

are adjudged ''safe and effective''—and effective means more than that they bring relief from a specified ailment. This relief must come from direct biological action on body processes and not simply from the placebo effect (although in actual use this effect may help greatly).

To produce direct therapeutic effects in the body, most drugs must get into the bloodstream. The majority are swallowed in the form of tablets, capsules or liquids, eventually being absorbed into the blood. Others are injected, applied to the skin, sniffed through the nose, placed under the tongue or inserted as suppositories into rectum or vagina. Once in circulation, the drug may work directly on cells of the ailing organ or tissue, combine with body chemicals to block disordered functions or restore healthy ones, or kill infectious microorganisms or cancer cells *(Chapter 4)*.

No drug produces just one effect in the body. Besides the desired therapeutic outcome, often called the primary effect, every medicine has one or more secondary effects that can be helpful, annoying or dangerous. Such secondary effects can arise from the drug alone or from a medicine's combining in the body with almost anything from aspirin to avocado.

Although most secondary actions are unwanted, some may enable one drug to relieve two quite different ailments—the effect that is secondary for one ill becomes primary for the other. And combinations of interacting substances can be used to increase the effectiveness of therapy. For example, two antimicrobials, trimethoprim and sulfamethoxazole, are sometimes used together because trimethoprim increases the other's actions against certain infections.

Weighing special risks

Both primary and secondary actions affect some people more than others, and the known patterns of such variations provide useful guides—and cautions for drug use. Weight, age, sex and state of general health are major influences. A standard dose of a drug, generally specified for someone who is between 18 and 65 years of age and weighs between 130 and 200 pounds, may be fine for the average man but a dangerous

A medical tragedy: the pitfalls of testing a wonder drug

When a German drug manufacturer, Chemie Grünenthal, first marketed a sedative called thalidomide in 1957, it called the medicine ''astonishingly safe.'' Later claims stated that the drug could ''be given with complete safety to pregnant women and nursing mothers, without adverse effect on mother or child.'' Over the next several years, however, in one of modern medicine's major tragedies, more than 7,000 European mothers—some of whom had taken as few as one or two thalidomide pills in pregnancy—bore malformed children. Most newborns were victims of a hitherto rare condition in which arms and legs were missing or consisted of flipperlike appendages extending from the torso.

Thalidomide had reached European markets on the strength of routine laboratory toxicity tests. The researchers gave the drug to adult rats, but not to pregnant rats. When it proved nonpoisonous to the test subjects, they concluded it was safe for humans.

That conclusion was challenged at the time by Dr. Frances O. Kelsey, a medical officer at the U.S. Food and Drug Administration. Dr. Kelsey believed that the research presented on thalidomide was insufficient, and she effectively blocked its sale in the United States.

More thorough research proved Dr. Kelsey right. In monkeys and baboons, whose reactions to certain drugs more closely resemble those of humans, the drug caused offspring to be born with stunted limbs. Pregnant rats exposed to the compound bore fewer young. That research—and the drug's withdrawal from the market in the early '60s—was scant consolation for the more than 7,000 who had suffered thalidomide's ravages.

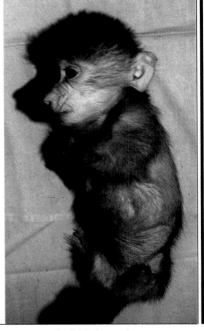

A two-week-old baboon, born to a female given thalidomide during pregnancy, suffers some of the defects the drug causes in humans: missing arm and leg bones and disfigured fingers.

overdose for a very frail elderly woman. In many cases doctors should calculate special doses for those who are extraordinarily under- or overweight, and of course for children. Other influences may not be so obvious, and anyone who has had experience with a given drug should advise the doctor if the dosage must be larger or smaller than usual.

Older people and those with debilitating illnesses run special risks of drug reactions. They may have digestive systems that will not absorb a drug properly, circulatory and nervous systems that may respond to it in unexpected ways, or impaired liver or kidney function that may restrict elimination and cause the drug to accumulate to a toxic level. As people age, moreover, they tend to take more medicines for various ailments, often from different doctors who may not know what the others are prescribing. Deafness, poor eyesight or arthritic fingers may complicate the simple act of following instructions in taking medicines. As a result, ill effects occur three times more often among the elderly than in the population as a whole.

Women also tend to have special problems with drugs. On the average, they go to doctors more frequently than men and receive more than one and a half times as many prescriptions. Thus they are exposed more to all the hazards of drugs. At certain times in the menstrual cycle, moreover, women of childbearing age produce higher levels of hormones, which may interact adversely with drugs.

Most important, a woman who is pregnant can pass on toxic, even deforming, chemicals to the fetus in her womb. The most tragic example was the disaster caused in the late 1950s and early 1960s by thalidomide *(opposite)*. A sedative thought to be safe, thalidomide was responsible for the deaths of thousands of infants and the births of thousands more with tragic deformities. The tragedy still hangs like a shadow over all drug use during pregnancy, particularly during the first three months, when the unborn baby develops not only limbs but also the major organs. Many drugs—even alcohol and tobacco—can cause irreparable harm then.

It is now known that if a woman has not yet discovered she is pregnant and takes an oral contraceptive early in the first three months of pregnancy, she may increase the risk of limb and heart defects in her infant. And it is a well-documented fact that women who take diethylstilbestrol to reduce the risk of a miscarriage may increase the risk of vaginal or cervical cancer later in the life of a female child. For this reason warnings are now required that any woman using birth-control pills stop taking them immediately and consult her physician if she thinks she is pregnant.

Other drugs to be avoided during pregnancy are antibiotics of the tetracycline group, which can cause permanent discoloration of children's teeth, and cortisone drugs used to relieve inflammation, which can damage developing adrenal glands. During the later stages of pregnancy, expectant mothers should not take anticoagulants and should use aspirin and similar salicylate compounds only very sparingly; these can prolong pregnancy and labor, can cause excessive bleeding at delivery, and may increase the risk of stillbirth. Also suspect are barbiturates, which can cause infants to be addicted before they are even born, and many kinds of tranquilizers, which may increase the risk of cleft lip.

For such reasons pregnant women are advised not to take drugs—any drugs—unless absolutely necessary, and then only on a doctor's advice. Because most drugs taken by a nursing mother will be present to some degree in her milk and thus will be passed on to her child, the same cautions apply to the use of medicines while breast feeding.

Balancing such risks against the often crucial benefits offered by modern drugs is easier if, whenever you must make the decision for yourself or your family, you consider one basic point: Do you need it? Do not use any more medicines than you absolutely have to; the more different drugs you take, the more likely you are to suffer an undesirable reaction or to have one drug interfere with or exaggerate the effects of another. If you find you must use nonprescription medicines for a persistent disorder—arthritis, recurrent headaches, stomach upsets—consult your doctor and your pharmacist.

How to get the most from any medicine

You will get the most out of any medicines you do need to take—and avoid mistakes—if you follow certain simple guidelines. Read the label of any medicine carefully before

In a Greek community in New York City, a woman pats heavy woolen socks soaked in ouzo—90-proof licorice-flavored cordial—on a man's stomach to demonstrate an old therapy for indigestion. The alcohol rapidly evaporates, cooling the skin; the feeling of chill helps block the sensation of internal pain.

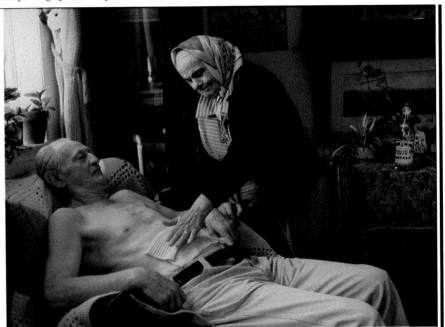

Folk remedies: They may help, and probably don't hurt

Every culture has its own stock of folk remedies, from the Slovak practice of wrapping horse-radish leaves around an aching head to the use by rural Louisiana blacks of filé—powdered sassafras leaves—as a palliative for burns. Many of these curatives are simple kitchen-cupboard supplies, but Greeks have taken up less common nonmedicinal substances such as the hearty cordial ouzo and cigarette ashes for the treatments shown here.

Often, the power of traditional cures lies with the patient's faith in their efficacy, especially when they are administered for an ill that, like most, would go away by itself. A few such remedies, however, seem to have a rational basis. Some researchers now believe that any part of the body can sustain only a limited amount of sensation, painful or pleasurable, at one time; so, by stimulating the distressed area with a different sensation, pain may diminish as the newly introduced feeling takes over. Thus, the tingle of horse-radish leaves or the cooling quality of filé is sufficient to make a patient feel the pain is being drawn out.

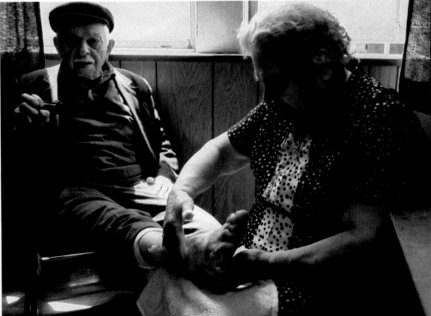

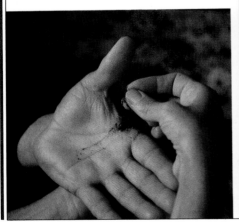

Cooled cigarette ashes were traditionally applied to cuts in an effort to promote healing as illustrated above. Although ashes have no proved antiseptic properties—and might even cause infection—they are believed to numb pain and stanch bleeding.

In a demonstration of a remedy for a sprain, a man's ankle is rubbed with hot, soapy water. The gentle massage might soothe the pain, but it could aggravate the swelling—cold packs are now known to be the best way to reduce inflammation. Because most minor sprains eventually heal themselves, however, the suds therapy was often given the credit for the cure.

you buy it—make sure you know exactly what it is, what it is meant to do, when and how to take it, what the proper dosage is and what precautions to observe. If there is anything you do not understand, ask your pharmacist. Each time you take a medicine, read the label again to make sure you have picked up the right one and that you are taking it at the right time and in the right amount.

If you are not getting relief from a medicine, do not take it more frequently than instructed or increase the dosage; another product or an entirely different treatment may be required. If you accidentally skip a dose, do not try to catch up by doubling the next dose; simply continue with the normal regimen and consult your physician. If you begin to feel well sooner than the doctor predicted or before you have taken as many pills as instructed, do not skip doses or stop. An antibiotic for a strep throat, for example, must be taken for some time after symptoms disappear, until all the guilty bacteria have been destroyed; otherwise, the survivors will spread again and bring back the symptoms.

If you need medicine at night, turn on the light; it is all too easy to confuse medicines in the dark or, when you are sleepy, to take a second and possibly dangerous dose of a drug you have already taken once. Do not keep medicines on a night table; force yourself to get up, and to wake up.

Keep a written record of all medicines—prescription drugs, vaccines, over-the-counter remedies—you take, noting unusual reactions to any drug so that it can be avoided in the future. Tell your doctor about these and make sure they are part of a permanent medical record, both at home and in your pharmacist's files *(Chapter 5)*. Buy only enough of a particular drug to last for the expected duration of the ailment. A week's supply of a cold remedy is ample: The symptoms seldom go on longer than that. In most households a bottle of 50 or 100 aspirin tablets is enough for occasional headaches and pains; keeping any more than that around gives long-unused pills a chance to deteriorate. Buying larger quantities may save money, however, if you must take the medicine regularly for relief from such chronic ailments as arthritis or high blood pressure.

Store all medicines according to the instructions on the label. If a label reads ''keep in a dry, cool place,'' try to find a place other than the bathroom medicine cabinet, which is apt to get steamy and warm. Most drugs can be stored at room temperature, as long as they are out of the sun. One of the worst places to put any medicine, even temporarily, is the glove compartment or trunk of an automobile, where temperatures can mount to 150° F., sometimes breaking down the chemical ingredients in a matter of hours.

Keep only those prescription medicines that you are currently using. Go through your stock once or twice a year and discard the medicines you seldom use and any whose expiration date—marked on the label—has passed. If there is any doubt about a medicine's identity, instructions for use or condition, throw it out.

Do not store medicines where young children can see or reach them, nor leave them on a bathroom counter or dressing table, even temporarily, if children are around. A bottle of pills left in a handbag is not much safer; it may take a child only a moment to find it and swallow enough to do serious harm. Although accidental poisonings have been greatly reduced by the packaging of drugs in child-resistant containers that cannot be opened without some feat of manual dexterity, the hazard has not been eliminated.

Never take medicines in front of children, or tell them a medicine tastes like candy or syrup to get them to take it. Popping pills while children are watching may trigger their natural tendency to imitate or make them think that those pretty little yellow, blue or pink pills must be taken by everyone who wants to be healthy and grown up.

Do not take a drug prescribed for anyone else (or give someone else a drug that was prescribed for you) even if the symptoms seem the same; there are many different disorders that have similar symptoms, and people differ in their reactions to the same drug.

The principal element in the prudent use of drugs is informed common sense. If you know what a medicine is meant to do—and not meant to do—you can choose drugs for simple ills yourself, buying them off the shelf. And you will be able to help your doctor and pharmacist give you the right prescriptions for the serious ills.   ❇

Feeding in their pens in a Utah dairy farm, these Holsteins are typical of the livestock that, when eventually slaughtered, provide the raw material for insulin used by two million diabetics in the United States. It takes about 8,000 pounds of pancreas from hogs and from dairy and beef cattle to yield one pound of pure insulin, but that is enough to supply 750 diabetics for a year.

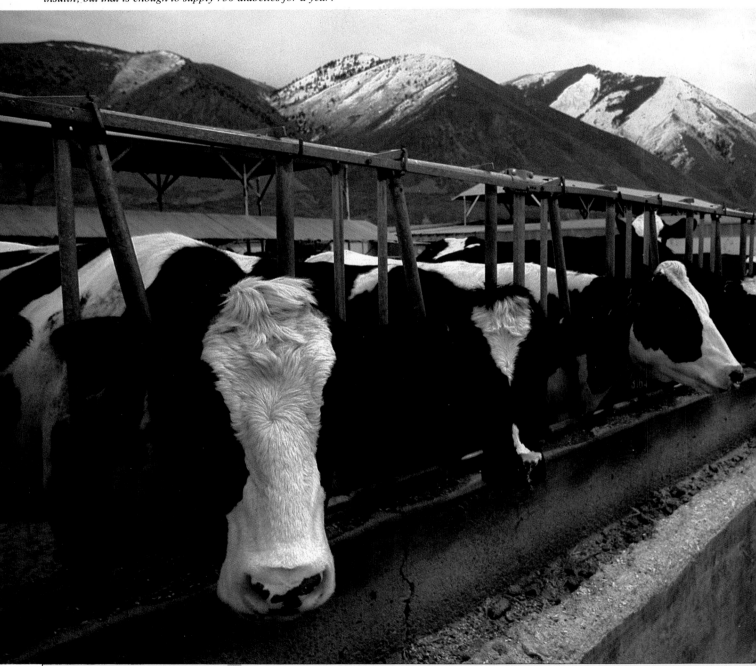

INSULIN PRODUCTION

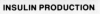

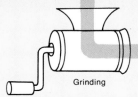
Grinding

Extraction

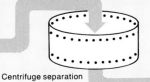
Centrifuge separation

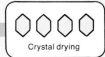
Crystal drying

Creating drugs from nature's bounty

"For every disease that afflicts mankind, there is a treatment or a cure occurring naturally on this earth," declared Norman R. Farnsworth of the University of Illinois. Farnsworth's faith has yet to be fully vindicated. But chemicals derived at least in part from plants, animals and microorganisms provide an estimated 40 per cent of prescription medicines. Indeed, the potential for obtaining medicines from natural sources is so great that thousands of substances are being studied for activity against such formidable foes as heart disease and cancer.

Among the best-known natural drugs is insulin, a hormone that regulates the blood's sugar content. People whose bodies cannot make insulin must have regular shots of the drug (below), prepared from the pancreas glands of cattle and swine. However, there is much more to producing insulin than conveying it from slaughterhouse to syringe. To make a medicine from a natural source—whether insulin from livestock pancreases or diosgenin for oral contraceptives from yams (pages 30-31)—requires a precise choreography of chemical operations. For insulin, the process—diagramed here in simplified form—takes eight months.

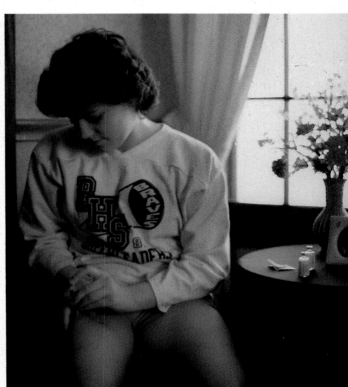

To make injectable insulin, pancreas glands are ground into a material resembling pink snow. It is mixed in an extraction tank with acidic alcohol to take insulin from the glands; the liquid is spun away from remaining solids in a centrifuge, a machine like a giant salad spinner. The alcohol is evaporated and salt added to crystallize the drug, which is then purified and dried.

A Minneapolis teenager stricken with diabetes starts the morning with the first of her two daily insulin injections. Combined with a strict diet and carefully regulated exercise, insulin enables her to live an active, relatively unhampered life.

A plant that can kill pain

From the seed pods of a poppy native to Turkey comes a painkiller whose potent effects were first noticed some 6,000 years ago: morphine. In its praise, the eminent Canadian physician Sir William Osler wrote: ''Morphine was God's own medicine.''

Morphine is one of several useful narcotic chemicals in the opium pod. In the extraction technique illustrated here—the ''poppy-straw concentrate'' method—morphine is obtained directly from dried pods, by-passing the production of opium. Another part of the pod—the seed—has no pharmacological value, but it is a favorite topping on bread and rolls.

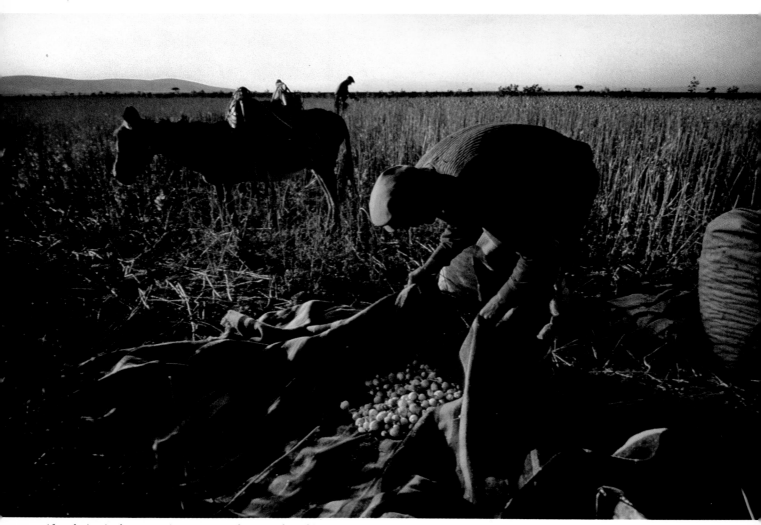

After drying in the sun, opium-poppy pods are gathered in bundles by a Turkish farmer who will transport them to market by donkey. The pods are purchased by a Turkish government agency, which oversees the extraction of unrefined morphine. Some 400 tons are shipped to U.S. drug firms annually.

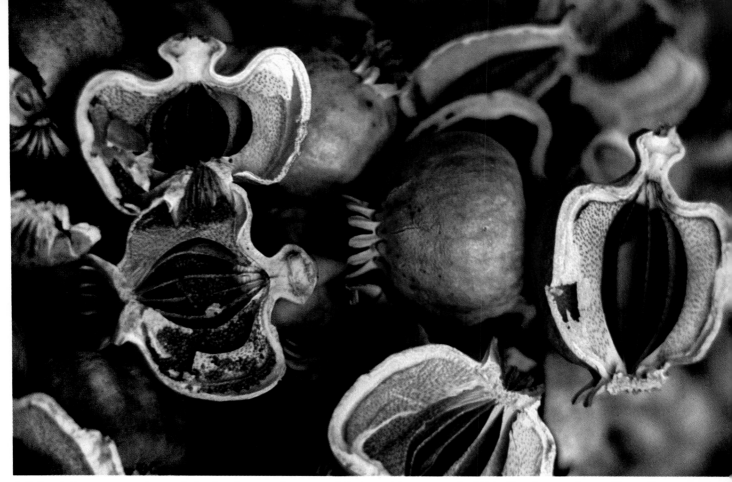

Split into halves, poppy pods—each the size of a tangerine—reveal the brownish centers and whitish skin where crude morphine collects.

MORPHINE PRODUCTION

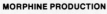

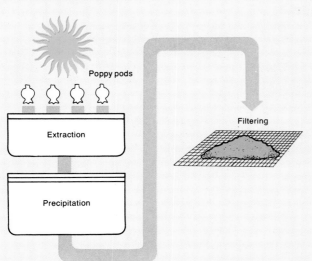

Sun-dried poppy pods—containing less than 1 per cent morphine—are dumped into an extraction tank of water, which dissolves the pods' active ingredients. After the liquid is concentrated, chemicals are added to adjust its acidity and initiate chemical changes that precipitate pure morphine crystals, which are then filtered out of the solution.

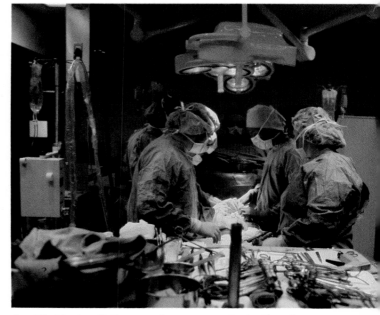

In a Washington, D.C., operating room a patient undergoing open-heart surgery is kept unconscious by morphine administered by an anesthesiologist (center, rear). Morphine, unlike other anesthetics, does not affect heart output or lower blood pressure, so it is often chosen for delicate heart operations.

In a flower bed in Texas, drug-company representatives monitor the growth of Madagascar periwinkles, whose leaf extracts provide the raw material for an anticancer drug. The plant grows wild in tropical Africa and on its namesake island. Huge quantities are needed for drug production—six or seven tons of leaves yield only an ounce of medicine.

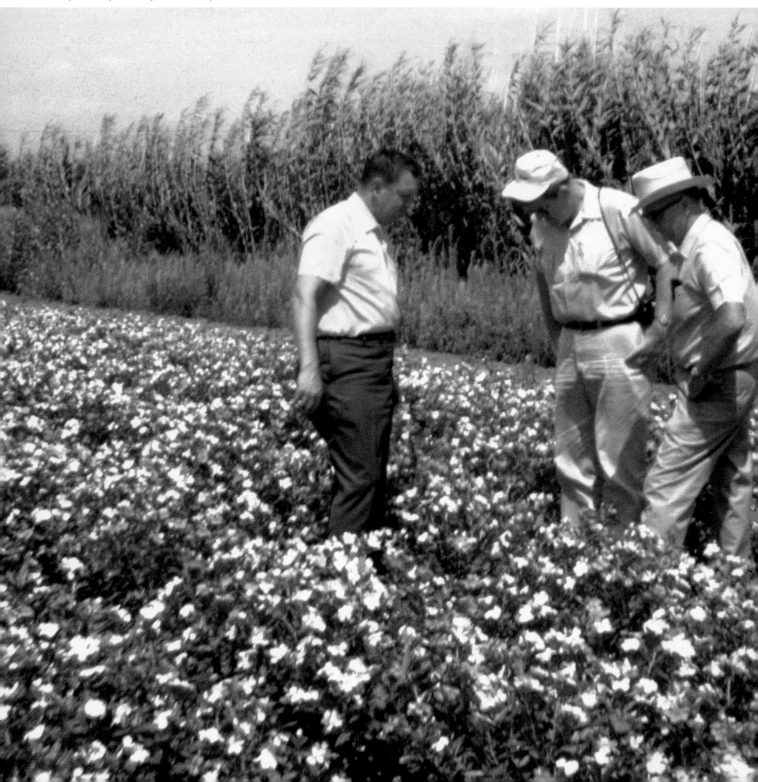

A flower that helps cure cancer

Some important new drugs are uncovered when medical investigators explore the territory of folk medicine—roots and leaves, herbs and other plants that local customs have sanctioned as cures. For example, the Madagascar periwinkle was tested in the 1950s for its supposed ability to control diabetes. The plant proved unusable for that condition, but it showed astonishing ability to fight some forms of cancer, particularly childhood leukemia, a disease of the blood-forming tissues. Further experiments yielded vincristine, a drug that helped make childhood leukemia, once inevitably fatal, curable in more than 50 per cent of the cases.

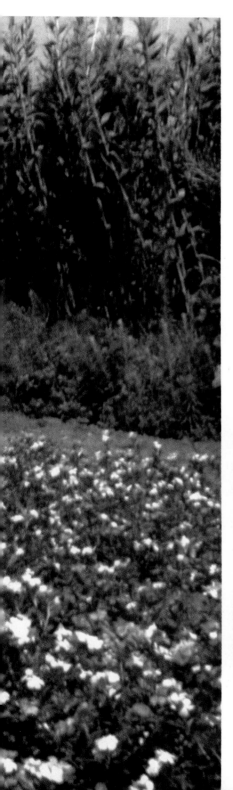

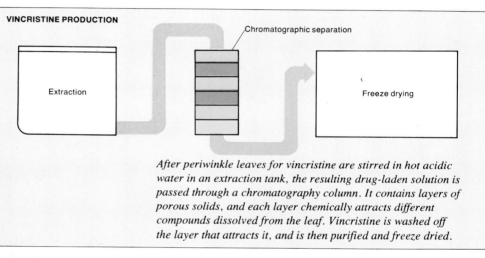

VINCRISTINE PRODUCTION

Chromatographic separation

Extraction

Freeze drying

After periwinkle leaves for vincristine are stirred in hot acidic water in an extraction tank, the resulting drug-laden solution is passed through a chromatography column. It contains layers of porous solids, and each layer chemically attracts different compounds dissolved from the leaf. Vincristine is washed off the layer that attracts it, and is then purified and freeze dried.

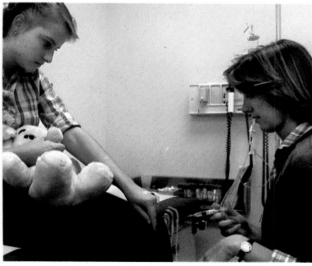

Clutching her stuffed elephant for security, a young leukemia victim offers her hand for an injection of vincristine. The drug is given as part of a regimen that includes several others.

A root that prevents conception

The revolutionary oral contraceptive called the Pill originated with an inedible jungle yam. Growing wild in Mexico, the yam had been used locally for centuries, but not for birth control. Its grated root was showered into lakes to stun fish for easy catching.

Studying the yam's chemical powers, Russell E. Marker, an American, found that it contains raw material for synthesizing many compounds that affect the human body—including male and female sex hormones, and cortisone, which promotes healing. One of those female hormones—estrone—when treated and refined, yielded the basic compound for oral birth-control drugs.

Clearing away a knot of vines, a farm worker prepares to detach the root of a wild Mexican yam that can be used to synthesize oral contraceptives and other compounds with medicinal applications.

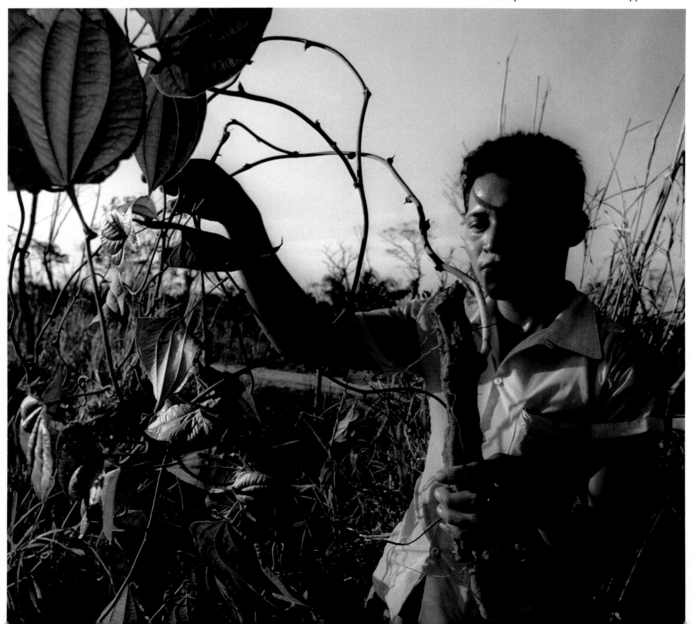

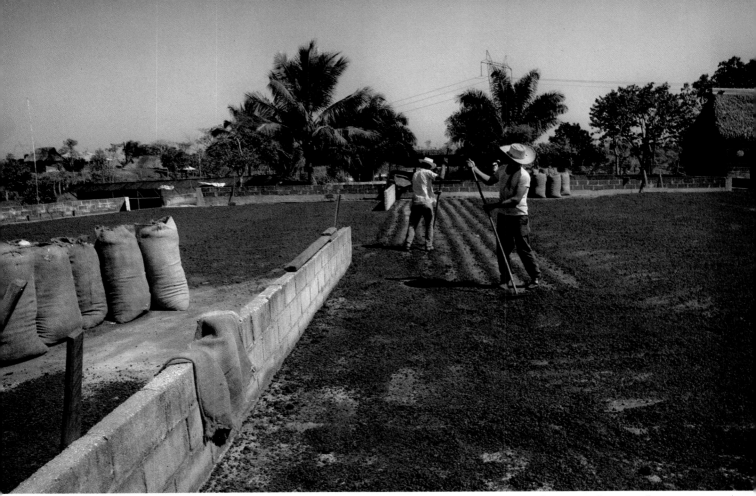

Drying in the Mexican sun, a thin layer of ground yam roots is raked into rows before being bagged for shipment to drug manufacturers.

ORAL-CONTRACEPTIVE PRODUCTION

Extraction

Molecular modification

Chilling

Boiling

In production of birth-control pills, ground yam roots are mixed in an extraction tank with a solvent that dissolves one of their active compounds, diosgenin. Treatments with heat and reagents rearrange the molecular structure of diosgenin into that of the female hormone estrone; it is combined with chemicals at −40° F. to produce norethindrone, which inhibits conception.

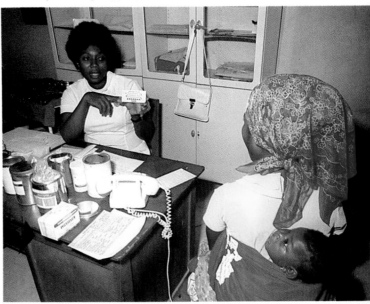

At a clinic in Ghana, a midwife explains the use of oral contraceptives to a woman with a child on her back. Birth-control pills are taken by more than 80 million women worldwide.

A fungus that fights infection

The worldwide search for microorganisms that yield germ killers has turned up slightly more than 60 that are of current value—one of the most significant of them a fungus scooped from a Sardinian gulf by Giuseppe Brotzu of the Institute of Hygiene at the University of Cagliari. Nearly two decades of arduous experiments and exacting molecular whittling were required in order to convert extracts from this sea life into a family of compounds, related to the penicillins, called cephalosporins. These compounds have proved to be effective against ailments ranging from staph infections to typhoid fever.

The picturesque waters of the Gulf of Cagliari, seen below from a fishing vessel floating off a Sardinian town, were the original source of the antibiotic fungus Cephalosporium. Today it is cultured in pharmaceutical laboratories.

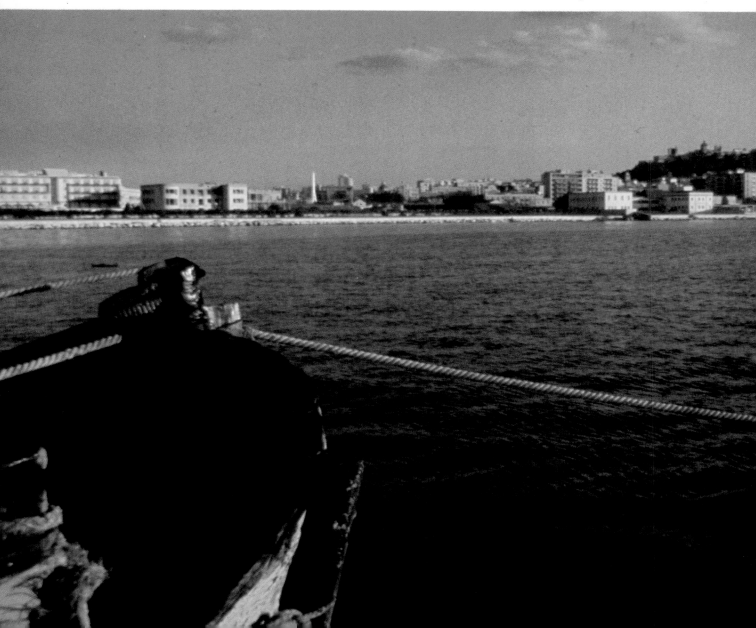

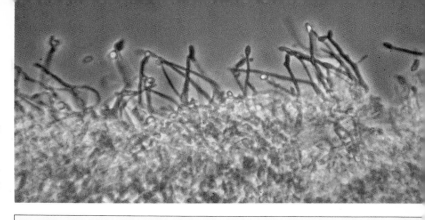

Magnified 160 times, Cephalosporium appears as a tangle of dark spindly stalks, each with an oval-shaped cap, surmounting a denser pattern of the microorganism's growth. It is grown on a food of lard oil, cornmeal or starch.

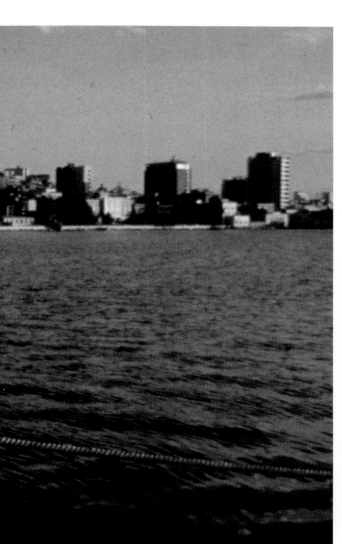

CEPHALOSPORIN PRODUCTION

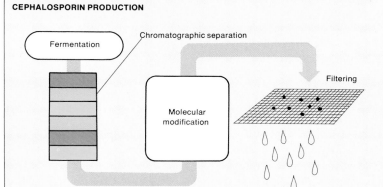

Fermentation

Chromatographic separation

Molecular modification

Filtering

Grown in a fermentation tank, Cephalosporium yields a solution containing an antibiotic, which is picked up by a resin layer in a chromatography column, washed off and then put through a series of chemical reactions. The result—depending on the way the cephalosporin molecule is modified—is one of several antibiotics in the form of a filtered powder.

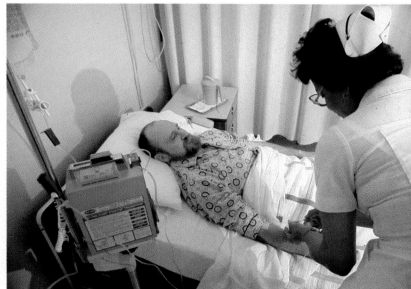

A man with a bacterial infection receives an injection of a newly developed variant of cephalosporin—cefamandole—from a nurse. One of a dozen cephalosporins now available, the drug was being tested for safety and effectiveness.

CHAPTER 2

The drugs you prescribe for yourself

Remedies recommended by the experts
Fast relief from pain
Treating the many symptoms of colds and flu
True cures for a sick stomach
Help for hemorrhoids
At last, skin remedies that work

In 1630 one Nicholas Knopp was sentenced by a Massachusetts Bay Colony court to be "fyned 5 pounds for takeing upon him to cure the scurvey by a water of noe worth nor value, which hee solde att a very deare rate, to be imprisoned till hee pay his fine or give securitye for it, or els be whipped & shall be lyable to any mans action of whom he hath receaved money for the said water."

Conditions have changed for the better since the days of Nicholas Knopp. The makers of nonprescription drugs who run afoul of the law no longer face the threat of a whipping, and most of their products have come to have considerable "worth and value"—more so since the early 1970s than in all the previous 340 years.

If improvement in easily obtained remedies was slow in coming, it was nonetheless welcome. According to the U.S. Department of Commerce, Americans diagnose three fourths of their own ailments and treat them with medicines bought without a prescription. They have to. There are not enough doctors, and probably never could be, to prescribe all the drugs that are needed. Simon Rottenberg, Professor of Economics at the University of Massachusetts, estimated that if just 2 per cent of the present users of nonprescription drugs were to consult doctors instead of making their own diagnoses, visits to doctors' offices would increase by more than 60 per cent; the medical profession would be overwhelmed.

Such self-prescription has long been essential, of course. It is much more effective today, partly because excellent, easy-to-use remedies have been developed for a large number of common ailments, and partly because new laws not only strengthen safeguards against dangerous medicines but also require that drugs be effective, able to relieve the conditions they claim they can treat. It was not always so. Even after the practice of medicine had acquired a scientific footing, around the end of the 19th Century, most makers of nonprescription drugs—also known as patent medicines—were still legally selling useless and sometimes dangerous nostrums, while making outrageous and baseless claims for their efficacy against all kinds of serious illnesses.

Many of those over-the-counter (or OTC) medicines could indeed make even a desperately ill patient feel better, at least for a while—their principal ingredients were alcohol, opium and opium derivatives such as morphine and heroin.

With passage of the Pure Food and Drugs Act of 1906 and establishment of what became the Food and Drug Administration (FDA), the federal government launched a long campaign to fight quackery and control narcotics in medicines. The government managed to drive off the market such patent medicines as Mrs. Winslow's Soothing Syrup, an infant-pacifier that the American Medical Association had called "a morphine-containing baby-killer," and Radam's Microbe Killer, which claimed to cure malaria, yellow fever, tuberculosis, smallpox and leprosy, although it was 99 per cent tap water and 1 per cent sulfuric and hydrochloric acid.

After the epidemic of gruesome birth defects caused by thalidomide *(page 20),* Congress in 1962 broadened the Food and Drug Administration's regulatory powers, laying the

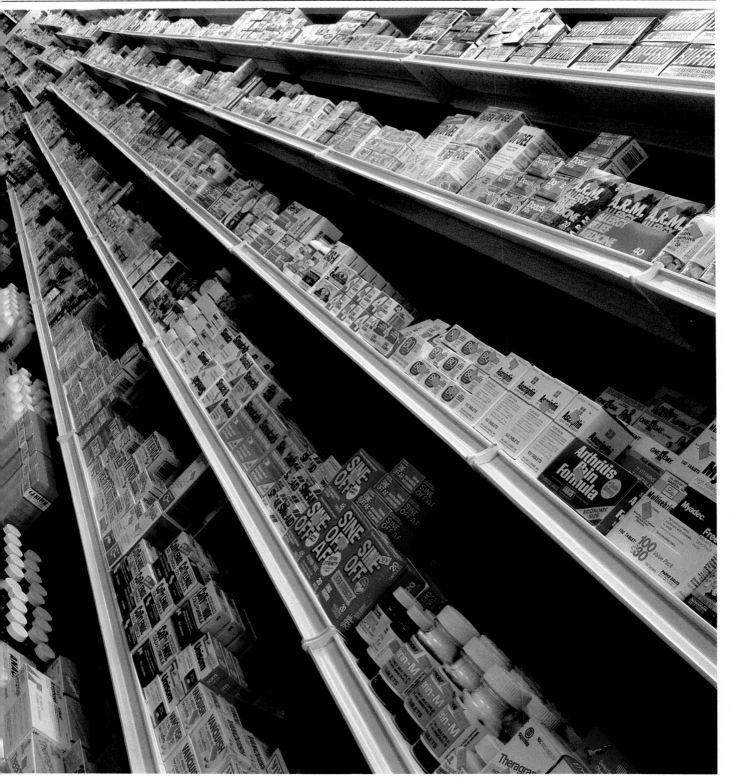

Hundreds of drugs, a tiny fraction of the quarter million or more nonprescription medicines available, cram the shelves of a discount drugstore. The self-service mass marketing of over-the-counter drugs is appropriate to their role in medicine: They are selected by the patients themselves, who diagnose their own illnesses—and they are used for three out of four ailments.

groundwork for a sweeping review of patent medicines. Beginning in 1972, the agency set out for the first time to investigate the safety and effectiveness of every single active ingredient in every over-the-counter drug on the market. Makers of medicines with unsafe ingredients would have to change their recipes or take the product off the market; products that were ineffective would have to be taken off the market; ingredients that did not contribute to a product's intended therapeutic effects would have to be eliminated from the recipe; manufacturers could not claim that their products accomplished more than was actually the case.

Remedies recommended by the experts

To accomplish this massive reexamination of medicines—including many that had been on the market for decades—the Food and Drug Administration created 17 panels, each made up of physicians, pharmacists, pharmacologists, re-search scientists, industry representatives and the public. The panels were organized in several ways. Some, such as the cough and cold panel, focused on ailments; others, such as the ophthalmic panel, on parts of the body. Still others, such as the laxative panel, were concerned with drug types.

Government officials optimistically predicted that the review would be completed in about three or four years, but after nine years much of the work remained to be done; the agency had seriously underestimated the size of the job. At the start of the review, officials believed that there might be some 200,000 products consisting of only 200 to 300 active ingredients. They were right to think that the basic ingredients numbered only a tiny fraction of the commercial products on the market. But their figures were wrong. By the end of 1979 the number of products had been tallied at over 250,000 and, more important, some 780 ingredients had been reviewed and the work was still going on.

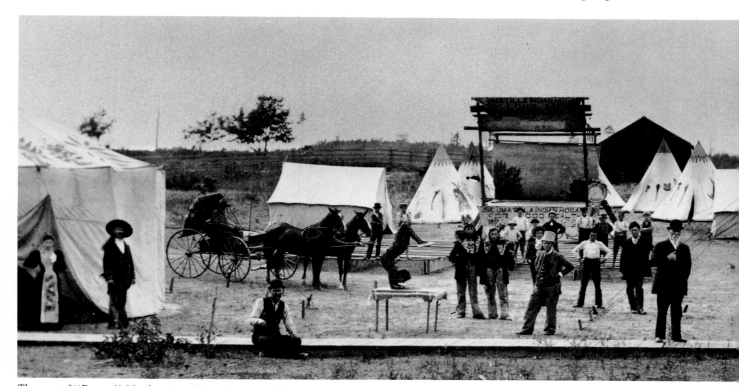

The cast of ''Doctor'' Matthews' medicine show, including stage Indians (center) and an acrobat (center left), pause between shows in the 1890s. This troupe, like most that promoted patent medicines, used entertainment to attract an audience for a sales pitch—to be delivered by the top-hatted doctor himself (far right), who touted a ''cure-all'' called Umatilla Indian Hogar.

After each drug has been reviewed, it is placed in one of three categories: Those in Category I are safe and effective for their indicated use; those in Category II are unsafe, ineffective or both and must be removed from the market; Category III drugs are those whose safety and effectiveness have not been decided, and they are allowed to stay on the market until the question is settled.

Although the process of banning a drug as ineffective can provoke lengthy court battles, several types of drugs have been swiftly barred from further sale for reasons of safety. One of these was the effective germ-killer known as hexachlorophene, used in deodorant soaps, shampoos and baby powders; it was removed from the over-the-counter market and made a prescription-only drug in 1972 when it was found to harm the nervous system in infants.

The claims made for other drugs have been sharply limited as a result of the review. For example, antihistamines, pro-

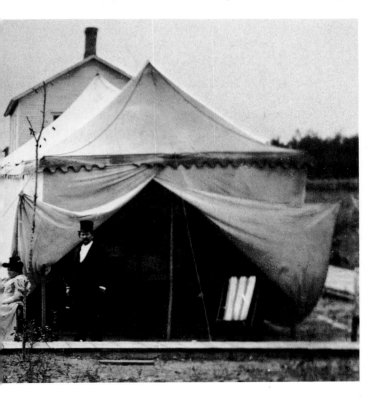

moted for the relief of nervous tension because they may cause drowsiness, can no longer be sold for that purpose, even though the same drugs can be marketed in nighttime sleep aids. The drowsiness produced by antihistamines was found by a panel to be dangerous in daytime use—and not helpful in relieving tension.

Such expert evaluation and rigid control would seem to eliminate all doubt about every container on a drugstore shelf. But anyone who expects to find only safe and certain remedies on sale expects too much. The quality of nonprescription drugs is much better than it was; it is not perfect and presumably will never be.

Many Category III drugs—those of questionable safety or efficacy—are on the market now, and considering the inexact nature of medical science, some of them will probably always be available. And many Category I drugs—accepted as safe and effective—are effective in only a minor way; alongside them on the drugstore shelf may be others that do the same job much better.

The most useful result of the official review of nonprescription drugs may be not governmental control over these remedies but the reports issued by the review panels. They contain information that serves as an invaluable guide in selecting drugs to treat a variety of common ills. The reports state unequivocally which medicines work. Their verdicts have been amplified by other authorities so that it becomes possible to identify not only which remedies work, but also which ones work best.

The reports of the review panels name names, but not, of course, brand names. The active ingredients are singled out, and they are identified by their generic chemical names. These terms may be lengthy and hard to pronounce, but they are the same ones that are listed on the labels of nonprescription medicines. Thus, once a recommended ingredient is known, it is fairly simple to check labels to find brands containing that ingredient.

Even the most specific guide to effective ingredients will not help in selecting a remedy unless the remedy can be matched to the sickness. Diagnosis often frustrates the experts, and self-diagnosis must be approached with great caution. Too many people die because they treat the pain of a heart attack with the medicine-chest cure for an upset stomach. Any symptom that is totally unfamiliar, recurs, causes severe pain or resists home remedies for several days signals the need of professional treatment.

Confidence that an ailment can be cured with a nonprescription drug is only the first step. Knowledge of one's own peculiarities and possible reactions to the drug is also necessary. The decongestants used to relieve cold symptoms, for example, can also cause an increase in blood pressure. Aspirin can cause excessive bleeding. Information about such side effects is generally on the drug label.

Thus self-prescription requires answers to three questions:
● Do the symptoms point to a serious illness or one that can be diagnosed and treated without the help of a doctor?
● If a doctor is not required, what over-the-counter medicine, if any, should be taken?
● Will the medicine cause any undesirable effects?

Although three out of four ills are treated without a doctor's help, a decision one way or the other must still be made in each case. Most problems not requiring professional help fall into one of four broad categories: first, minor pains such as headaches and muscle and joint aches; second, cold and flu discomforts; third, digestive upsets; and finally, skin afflictions. These are the ailments for which the widest selection of useful medicines is available without prescription and for which the official review panels, professional associations and other experts have provided the clearest guidance.

Fast relief from pain

The most common ill, and the most readily cured, is pain. Over-the-counter painkillers, particularly aspirin and its principal substitute, acetaminophen, will usually bring relief from minor aches in about 45 minutes. They work against nearly all headaches, muscle pains, toothaches and even pain caused by minor surgery such as dental repair. Aspirin—but not acetaminophen—also alleviates arthritis pain. Of course, aches can be symptoms of anything from an ulcer to a brain tumor, and even certain kinds of headaches, such as migraines and so-called cluster headaches, are serious ail-

ments in their own right, totally beyond the reach of any medicine available over the counter.

The ability of aspirin or acetaminophen to stop most simple aches, combined with their inability to cure pains that have more serious causes, gives the sufferer a basis for accurate diagnosis. If the drugstore remedy works, the problem is solved; if it does not, or if the ache returns and persists for several days, the problem is beyond the powers of nonprescription painkillers and it is time to see a doctor.

Aspirin—acetylsalicylic acid—gave the world a miraculous cure for pain at the height of patent-medicine quackery, but only after its value had gone unrecognized for half a century. Aspirin was first synthesized in 1853 by the Alsatian chemist Charles-Frédéric Gerhardt. He based his synthesis on salicylic acid, which was originally derived from the bark of the willow tree and was well known to ancient civilizations as a source of relief from pain. But neither Gerhardt—who regarded his invention simply as a chemical curiosity—nor anyone else over the following decades thought of using acetylsalicylic acid as a pain medicine. While that formula languished, the drug most commonly used for pain relief was salicylic acid—reasonably effective but so harsh that it frequently resulted in severe stomach upset.

Only when the father of Felix Hoffmann, a chemist at Friedrich Bayer and Co. in Elberfeld, Germany, asked his son to find him a milder analgesic for his arthritis was acetylsalicylic acid tried. The results were outstanding—the drug was easy to tolerate and strikingly effective in reducing pain. In the first few years of the 20th Century aspirin came into widespread use as a headache remedy and general painkiller, and its remarkable ability to reduce fever and inflammation was also demonstrated.

Aspirin is so effective that even the most imaginative advertiser would find it hard to exaggerate what it can do for simple headaches. It is, in the words of the television commercials, ''the ingredient doctors recommend most for headaches'' and ''the leading pain-relieving ingredient.'' When aspirin came up in the government-sponsored review of nonprescription drugs, its effectiveness was never in doubt.

The reviewers did, however, raise a question about dos-

The rise and fall of patent medicines

America in the 19th Century abounded with patent medicines, guaranteed by their makers to cure not only known diseases but such vague complaints as a "systemic catarrh" and an "impure state of the blood." Actually, the term "patent medicine" was misleading. Only the names of these nostrums were patented—and the so-called medicines were loaded with so many dangerous ingredients that the public eventually turned against them.

In their heyday the patent-medicine men proved, at least, that they were magnificent salesmen, with advertising campaigns that made their products familiar to anyone who ventured outdoors. Brightly colored posters filled shop windows, bigger-than-life signs covered the sides of barns, hawkers thrust leaflets into the hands of passersby, and armies of men marched the streets in sandwich signs proclaiming the virtues of patent medicines.

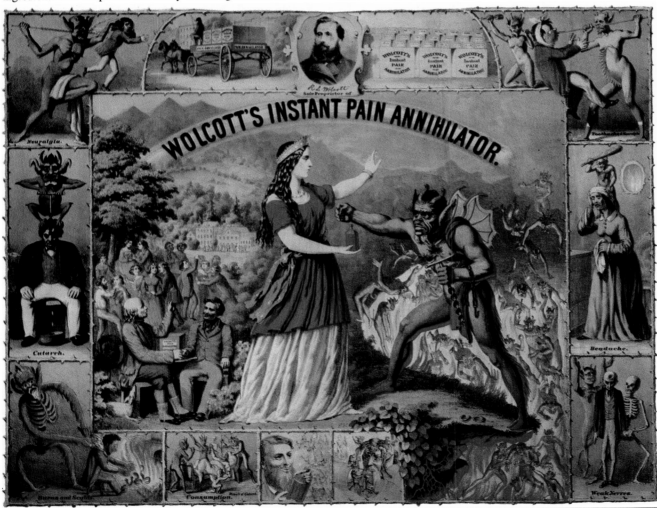

A martial maiden banishes the demon pain with a bottle of Wolcott's Annihilator while satisfied customers form a panorama of good health. The allegorical border typifies the extravagant claims made for patent medicines—this painkiller was not only aimed at such obvious targets as headaches, but was also supposed to cure tuberculosis and an ailment called weak nerves.

Mixes of herbs and deadly drugs

In *The Adventures of Tom Sawyer,* a naïve spinster samples a patent painkiller—the effect, according to author Mark Twain, was that of "fire in liquid form." It was probably a fair description. Most of these potions contained alcohol—sometimes as much as in 80-proof whiskey. Many used such dangerous narcotics as morphine and cocaine.

But the bottle labels, like the advertisements on these pages, rarely listed such potent ingredients; instead, the manufacturers generally touted their wares as mysteriously effective herbal mixtures. Unsuspecting consumers used the remedies in blithe ignorance of their contents, and some manufacturers audaciously sold their habit-forming drugs as cures for alcohol and drug addiction.

In an 1860 poster, a buckskin-clad frontiersman revives an emaciated settler with Ginger Brandy from a well-stocked saddlebag. Any restorative powers of the beverage came less from its ginger than from its high alcohol content.

Motherly love is the theme of an advertising card for a syrup that soothed crying infants—with morphine. Under government pressure, "Mrs. Winslow"— the real manufacturers were two brothers named Curtis—eventually reduced the amount of narcotic in the elixir.

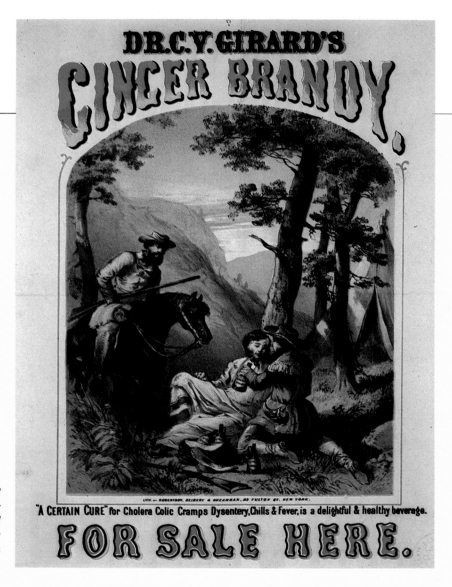

DR.C.V. GIRARD'S GINGER BRANDY.

"A CERTAIN CURE" for Cholera Colic Cramps Dysentery, Chills & Fever, is a delightful & healthy beverage.

FOR SALE HERE.

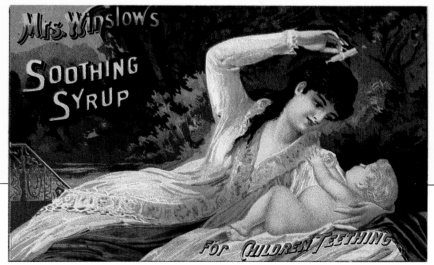

Mrs. Winslow's SOOTHING SYRUP

FOR CHILDREN TEETHING

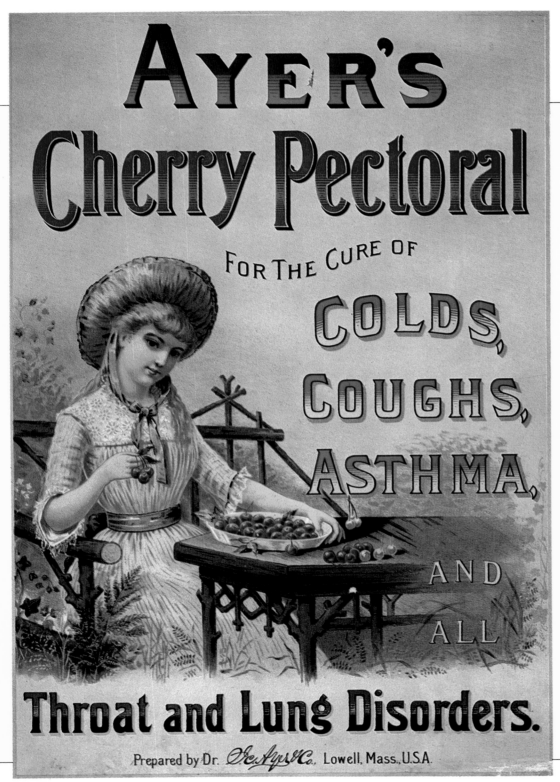

A beguiling picture and a misleading name suggest that Ayer's Pectoral somehow cures chest diseases by the healing power of a bowl of cherries. The preparation did contain some cherry flavoring, but its active ingredient was heroin.

The crusade against a "shameful trade"

In 1905, at a time when so-called muckraking journalists were exposing corruption in business and government, Samuel Hopkins Adams, writing for *Collier's* magazine, set out on a crusade against the evils of patent medicines. Calling worthless and harmful nostrums "the great American fraud," Adams blamed the injury to the public not only on producers, but also on "advertising bunco men." He called the industry a "shameful trade," and he thundered: "Every man who trades in this market takes toll of blood."

Adams' articles appeared at the right moment; for years, Americans had been growing increasingly aware of the menace in fake remedies. In 1906 Congress passed the Pure Food and Drugs Act, which permitted the sale of narcotics as medicine but required the labeling of all dangerous ingredients. Even under this early, limited legislation, many nostrums were forced off the market; for the remainder, manufacturers either altered the formulas or rewrote the labels.

"Death's Laboratory," an advertising cartoon for Collier's magazine, promotes Samuel Adams' magazine articles on the patent-drug industry. In this medley of symbols, a grotesque skull leers malevolently, with barrels of alcohol and narcotics nestled in its eyes and bottles of medicines forming its teeth. The shadowy creature filling the bottles is a bitter parody of the glamorous women featured in patent-medicine advertisements.

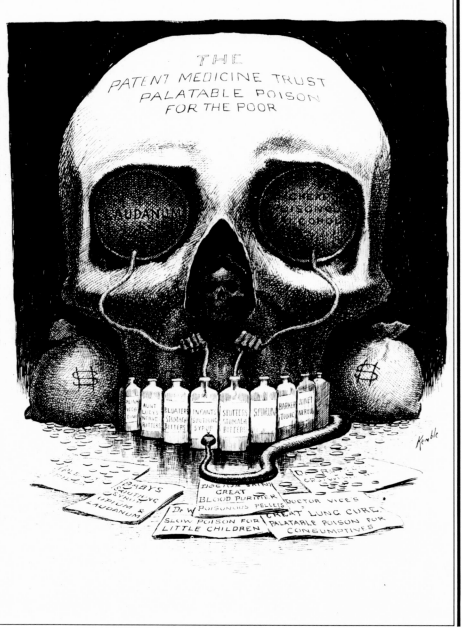

age. They recommended that it be sold only in pills containing 325 milligrams (often expressed as five grains, the grain being an ancient apothecary's measure based on the average weight of a grain of wheat and equivalent to 64.8 milligrams). They ruled against "maximum strength" tablets of 400 milligrams or more. Multi-ingredient drugs with less than 325 milligrams of aspirin also met with disapproval. The experts singled out the 325 milligram size as best because it is the minimum considered effective in adults, and it is easily doubled—two tablets—to give the maximum dose recommended. Aspirin doses of more than 650 milligrams without a doctor's supervision may create unnecessary risks. Timed-release versions of aspirin—capsules containing tiny pellets that disintegrate at different rates to spread the dosage over a longer time period—were also questioned since individual digestive systems may influence rates of absorption.

Although aspirin is as safe as it is effective for most people, it causes side effects that may be annoying—such as a ringing in the ears—or serious. It retards blood clotting, enough so that doctors have begun using it to prevent the clotting that can lead to strokes and heart attacks—but also enough to be dangerous for anyone already taking anticoagulants, for patients scheduled for surgery, or for a pregnant woman about to give birth.

Because aspirin is an acid, it irritates the stomach, causing nausea in as many as 10 per cent of users. If the irritation is not serious, it can be avoided by taking the drug with milk or solid food or by using painkillers that combine aspirin with an antacid. However, aspirin can precipitate an ulcer attack in those susceptible to this ailment, and if the ulcer bleeds, aspirin's anticoagulant effect will worsen the bleeding.

People who cannot tolerate aspirin at all need not suffer without relief. Among the several aspirin substitutes, only one—acetaminophen—was considered both safe and fully effective. Acetaminophen works as well as aspirin for headaches and other pains, and without aspirin's gastric and allergic side effects. But this drug can cause kidney and liver damage if taken in large amounts, so it is vital to carefully follow the label's dosage instructions. And unlike aspirin, acetaminophen does not relieve soreness that comes with

inflammation, a condition—as in arthritis—signaled by redness, heat and swelling.

Brand-name medicines offering aspirin and acetaminophen in combination are not as effective as either drug alone; nor does caffeine, combined with aspirin in several painkiller brands, make them more effective.

Among the many other nonprescription painkillers, several types were found to be of some value. Local anesthetics such as benzocaine, phenol or butacaine help relieve sore gums, and a medicine called eugenol helps toothaches. Similarly, liniments, gels, lotions and ointments provide some relief for ordinary muscle and joint aches, whether caused by a cold, overexertion, arthritis, or nerve malfunction. These salves contain solutions of such materials as camphor, thynol, turpentine oil, mustard, menthol and salicylate compounds—related chemically to aspirin—that, when rubbed briskly into the skin, mildly irritate the area and provoke a warm, soothing reaction. However, according to the American Pharmaceutical Association, aspirin and—except in the case of arthritis—acetaminophen may do these jobs better.

Treating the many symptoms of colds and flu

Without peers against aches and pains, aspirin and acetaminophen are also major weapons in the struggle against two other unavoidable and bothersome ailments—the common cold and influenza. Both illnesses are viral infections of the breathing passages in the head and throat. Because viruses burrow inside human cells and stay there, antibiotics cannot reach and destroy them and therefore cannot cure these infections. They must run their course, the average cold lasting about a week, flu up to several weeks. But if no medicine can cure them, several over-the-counter medicines—most relying mainly on aspirin or acetaminophen—are effective against the sometimes painful symptoms.

The most heavily advertised cold and flu products take aim—often faulty aim—at a great many symptoms at once. The multi-ingredient, or "shotgun," remedies pitched so relentlessly as a cure for the multiple discomforts of a cold are based on a sound premise: Cold sufferers do experience many symptoms. According to the American Pharmaceutical

Association's *Handbook of Nonprescription Drugs*, 100 per cent of cold victims get a runny nose; almost as many suffer stuffiness, sneezing and a sore or dry throat; three quarters or more have postnasal drip, headache and cough, and a general feeling of malaise; almost half have fever and chills; and 20 per cent or more experience body aches and burning eyes.

Such overwhelming numbers would seem to make a strong case for use of shotgun remedies. But the percentages create a mathematical illusion. Only one cold sufferer in 200 is apt to have all 12 symptoms, and even the eight symptoms that, separately, occur in three quarters or more of cold victims will be combined in only about one sufferer out of three.

One multipurpose remedy is valuable—it can relieve headaches, the pain of stuffed-up sinuses, fever and chills, body aches and sore throat. But this miraculous product is hardly a shotgun remedy. More like a single bullet, it is the almighty aspirin tablet or its substitute, acetaminophen.

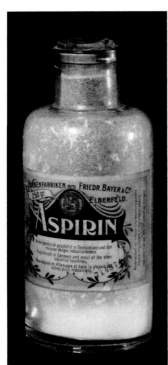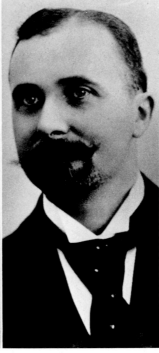

The formidable pain-relieving power of aspirin was discovered in the 1890s by the German chemist Felix Hoffmann, who had been seeking a medicine to allay his father's rheumatism. Until a method was devised about 1915 to produce aspirin in tablet form, it was sold as a powder (left).

Although both painkillers have a sovereign effect against the fevers and accompanying chills that hit about half of all cold sufferers, doctors disagree on their use for this purpose. Some authorities believe that unless fever rises above 105° in an adult, threatening brain damage, aspirin or acetaminophen should not be used in most cases. They recommend that fever be left alone because it may help overcome the infection—it seems to be involved in natural defenses against disease. However, most physicians believe these curative effects are marginal and are outweighed by the relief to be gained from reducing the fever.

No such dispute surrounds the use of standard pain-killers for sore throat, although other, more or less soothing treatments are available. Gargling may bring relief, but no nonprescription gargle medicine is better than warm water and salt, and preparations containing antiseptics can make the throat drier and sorer. Sucking hard candy may help, as will over-the-counter lozenges containing concentrations of from 5 to 20 per cent of the local anesthetic benzocaine. But if the sore throat is severe enough to interfere with normal activities, only a medicine prescribed by a doctor will be potent enough to ease the pain by removing its underlying cause—in many cases the bacterial infection known as strep throat.

As versatile as aspirin and acetaminophen are against many of the miseries of colds and flu, illnesses such as these may require more than a painkiller. A runny, stopped-up nose and burning eyes plague most cold and flu sufferers, and there are some very effective medicines to help ease these discomforts. But which medicine to use depends on whether the symptoms are caused by cold or flu virus or by an allergy. The symptoms for both are similar, yet what works effectively against an allergy does not work against a virus.

Most people distinguish between these two causes of similar symptoms from personal experience. Watery eyes, a runny and itchy nose, and an attack of repetitive sneezing following exposure to such substances as pollen or dust are signs of allergy, particularly if the aches and malaise of a virus attack are absent. The allergic reactions appear when the body releases chemicals called histamines, which swell the blood vessels around the nasal passages and inflame the mucous membrane that lines the passages. The action of the histamines can be countered by antihistamines, chemicals with such jawbreaking names as brompheniramine maleate, chlorpheniramine maleate, and doxylamine succinate.

Antihistamines have nothing more than a slight drying effect on the sniffling and sneezing of a cold or flu because these viral symptoms are caused not primarily by the release of histamines but by other defense reactions of the body. The cold or flu congestion requires something that counters these reactions—a decongestant, or a vasoconstrictor, which serves to shrink the swollen blood vessels. In addition, however, decongestants may aggravate such ailments as hyperthyroidism, high blood pressure, heart disease and diabetes. Decongestants may also act on the nervous system, causing jumpiness and insomnia.

Some of the most widely advertised cold remedies contain decongestants; unfortunately, many of them also contain antihistamines, which serve little or no purpose. Many also include antacids, presumably for the few users bothered by the aspirin in the potion, and some even have caffeine to counteract the drowsiness caused by the antihistamines. It is better, the review panel indicated, to treat cold or flu sniffles with a drug that is simply a decongestant, rather than attack it with a combination of many ingredients.

Decongestants can be swallowed in the form of pills or applied to inner nasal surfaces in the form of sprays, drops, gels or inhalants. The pills, as their ingredients circulate through the body, can introduce severe side effects. They are also relatively less effective than many types that are applied directly to the mucous membrane—the topical decongestants. Among the topical decongestants, gels rank second to other types because they may not penetrate mucous blockage to get to the surfaces most troubled by congestion. Sprays can penetrate nasal obstructions, as do drops, but sprays cover a larger area. Any of the topical decongestants can be overused—taking them for more than four days can cause irritation that stimulates more congestion than it clears up, a condition known as nasal rebound. If the victim resorts to further use of the drug, he may damage the mucous membrane or become dependent on the medicine in order to breathe easily.

One of the most widely used of the decongestant compounds judged acceptable by the review panel is phenylephrine. Other acceptable ingredients are naphazoline—more potent and more irritating to the nasal surfaces than phenylephrine—and oxymetazoline and xylometazoline, which are longer-lasting. Also used are phenylpropanolamine and pseudoephedrine, available only in pills.

When and how to quiet a cough

The one symptom of a cold or flu that cannot be reached by painkillers or decongestants is the cough. The specific remedy, called a cough suppressant, is omitted from most of the cold remedies, no matter how many other drugs are included in their shotgun blasts. On the other hand, virtually all of the products that are sold as cough suppressants do include ingredients that are found in most cold medicines but have nothing to do with suppressing a cough.

Cough suppressants work by desensitizing the cough reflex in the brain. The most effective is the opium derivative known as codeine. As a narcotic, codeine is strictly regulated by federal law and is available only in small concentrations in a few over-the-counter cough syrups. Many states prohibit codeine in any nonprescription medicine.

Only one non-narcotic cough suppressant was found to be an effective substitute for codeine: a nonaddictive, synthetic opiate called dextromethorphan. It is available in pills and syrups in every state.

Even though coughs can readily be suppressed, not all of them should be. Doctors generally agree on the benefits of stopping a dry cough, one that does not eject mucus and other matter into the throat and mouth. However, a productive cough that brings up material to be spit out serves the useful purpose of ridding the respiratory system of harmful substances. Most doctors say that productive coughs should not be suppressed; but some would make an exception for severe coughing that noticeably weakens the patient or prevents him from getting a good night's sleep.

Productive coughs are helped by liquefying the sputum so that the cough does its ejecting job better. A great many cough remedies on the market contain various drugs, called

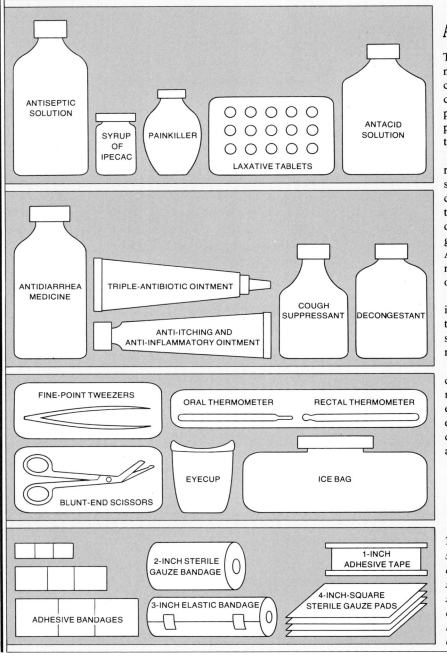

ANTISEPTIC
SOLUTION

SYRUP
OF
IPECAC

PAINKILLER

LAXATIVE TABLETS

ANTACID
SOLUTION

ANTIDIARRHEA
MEDICINE

TRIPLE-ANTIBIOTIC OINTMENT

ANTI-ITCHING AND
ANTI-INFLAMMATORY OINTMENT

COUGH
SUPPRESSANT

DECONGESTANT

FINE-POINT TWEEZERS

ORAL THERMOMETER

RECTAL THERMOMETER

BLUNT-END SCISSORS

EYECUP

ICE BAG

ADHESIVE BANDAGES

2-INCH STERILE
GAUZE BANDAGE

3-INCH ELASTIC BANDAGE

1-INCH
ADHESIVE TAPE

4-INCH-SQUARE
STERILE GAUZE PADS

A kit for the home doctor

To take care of everyday injuries and ill-nesses, the home doctor needs a medicine-cabinet kit like the one sketched at left. It contains nonprescription medicines and sim-ple instruments and supplies to treat medical problems that do not require professional at-tention—and most do not.

For minor wounds, there are tweezers to remove splinters or glass fragments, an anti-septic solution such as iodine to disinfect cuts, and a triple-antibiotic ointment to pro-tect wounds against infection. Adhesive ban-dages seal small cuts; pads and rolls of sterile gauze bandage are used for larger wounds. Adhesive tape and blunt-end scissors are also needed to secure the bandages and to prepare or remove the dressings.

For sprains, an ice bag will reduce swell-ing immediately after an injury, and an elas-tic bandage will both immobilize and support sprained or dislocated parts. An eyecup helps rinse irritants from the eyes.

Syrup of ipecac, which induces vomiting in cases of poisoning, is included because it must be on hand for immediate use in an emergency. Caution: Ipecac must not be used except on the advice of a physician or poison-control center; in some cases, the syrup could aggravate the effects of the poison.

The home medical supplies shown in this sketch should not be stored in the bathroom cabinet, as they often are. Rather, they should be kept out of children's reach in a separate, lockable cupboard or drawer or on a high shelf in an adult's bedroom. Medicines should be protected from bright light, extreme heat or high humidity.

expectorants, that are supposed to accomplish this goal. The review panel was not convinced that any of them works. And irrationally, many are mixed with a cough suppressant. For the productive cough, no medicine does as much good as moist air in a humidified room.

True cures for a sick stomach

If the causes of colds and flu are known but intractable—only the symptoms can be alleviated—the opposite is true of the common ills that afflict the digestive system. Indigestion, nausea, constipation, diarrhea or hemorrhoids arise from multiple sources, many of them mysterious, but most of these ailments can be cured with simple medications.

Indigestion, whatever its fundamental cause, strikes when the body secretes an excess of digestive fluids—primarily hydrochloric acid—irritating the stomach lining. The resulting discomfort in the upper abdomen is often described as sour stomach or heartburn.

Literally thousands of products are available to neutralize this excess acid and settle the stomach. But making up that multitude of brands are but four common active ingredients: sodium bicarbonate (better known by its old-fashioned name, bicarbonate of soda), calcium carbonate, magnesium salts and aluminum salts. Two act rapidly but have a relatively short-lived effect, while the other two are slower-acting but longer-lasting. And any of these formulated as liquid will work better than tablets.

One fast-acting drug is sodium bicarbonate. Though ordinarily quite safe, it contains sodium, an element that raises blood pressure and is not recommended for those suffering from high blood pressure or heart disease. The other fast-working antacid is calcium carbonate. Occasionally, however, this drug may cause the stomach to overcompensate, producing an even greater excess of acid—acid rebound.

The other two approved antacids are slower and more persistent, requiring about an hour to take effect. Oddly, aluminum compounds can cause constipation and those of magnesium can cause diarrhea, so the two are often sold as a combination in which the side effects cancel each other out.

If acid indigestion is accompanied by nausea, an antacid will help both ills. Only one other form of nausea, motion sickness, is affected by nonprescription drugs. It arises when the rolling movements of a boat, car or airplane disturb the balance organ in the inner ear, and it can be prevented by any of the drugs that limit that organ's sensitivity: meclizine, cyclizine and dimenhydrinate. They work most effectively as preventives. Plan to take the initial dose of meclizine an hour before the beginning of a trip; give either of the other two at least a half hour's head start. Meclizine is extremely long-lasting, one dose being sufficient for 24 hours, but it should never be used for children under the age of 12. The other two drugs can be taken up to four times a day and they are safe for children if taken in smaller doses.

More general help is available for diarrhea, which occurs when the digestive system works too fast, giving the intestines insufficient time to absorb water from the food and drink passing through. Diarrhea can result from excesses of eating, drinking and smoking that cause bowel irritation. It can be triggered by a brief bacterial infection of the digestive system—the misnamed "24-hour flu" or "intestinal flu." Occasionally, it results from a bacterial imbalance caused by antibiotics, by tainted food or by unfamiliar bacteria in food and water eaten away from home.

A large number of nonprescription antidiarrhea agents are for sale, but only two were approved by the government reviewers. One is opium—in the time-honored form of paregoric, which slows the action of the intestines, giving them time to soak up more water. But because paregoric is a narcotic, many states ban it for sale without a prescription, even in the low concentrations permitted by federal law. The only other effective nonprescription treatment for diarrhea is polycarbophil, an absorbent that draws up about 60 times its weight in water but is otherwise totally inert.

Strangely, polycarbophil is also effective against that opposite ailment, constipation. But for this purpose, polycarbophil is only one of several over-the-counter medicines that are safe and effective. The question to be posed is not whether they work but whether and when they are needed. Americans' concern for regularity flies in the face of medical opinion. According to a text on the subject by Dr. Horace W.

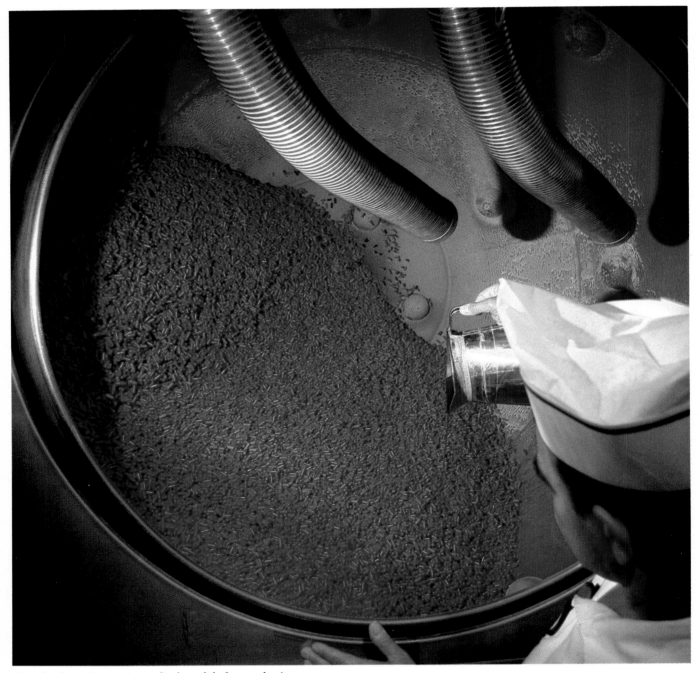

A batch of vitamins receives a final touch before packaging—a crimson covering solution poured on by a factory worker. Hot air then courses through the corrugated tubes to speed the drying process. Coatings may be used to improve taste and appearance, protect ingredients from air and moisture, and prevent the drug from dissolving until it has been swallowed.

Davenport of the University of Michigan Medical School, three times a day or once a week can be as normal as a daily bowel movement for different, equally healthy individuals.

When constipation becomes bothersome, it can often be cured by changing a diet to include more liquids, and foods high in fiber, such as whole fruit, vegetables and bran cereals; these substances provide more of the bulk and moisture needed for elimination. For faster relief, treatments work differently. Fastest of all are suppositories and enemas. Concentrated salt solutions, such as magnesium hydroxide, better known as milk of magnesia, are thought to cause the body to add fluid to the intestines to get rid of the salts. Stimulants goad the lower digestive system into faster and more vigorous action. Effective stimulants include senna, cascara, phenolphthalein, bisacodyl and danthron.

Gentler, slower-acting laxatives, which take 12 to 24 hours to work, are either bulk-forming laxatives or emollients, also called stool-softeners, both of which increase the amount of water in the stool. Effective bulk-forming laxatives include methylcellulose, psyllium, and polycarbophil, the substance that works equally well against diarrhea and constipation. The stool-softeners are docusate sodium, docusate calcium and docusate potassium.

The review panel on laxatives recommended that the fast-acting stimulant and saline drugs and the slower-acting stool-softeners and lubricants should be used only occasionally and for no longer than a week. In cases of stubborn constipation with no indication of serious underlying causes, the bulk-forming laxatives are preferable because they are inert, and ordinarily do not affect the digestive processes. They should be taken with a full glass of water. Mineral oil, a traditional home remedy for constipation, was approved by the panel but is objected to by many physicians: It may prevent the absorption of certain vitamins, and it may also be absorbed into the lungs, causing a form of pneumonia.

Help for hemorrhoids

Constipation can be an aggravating factor in the burning, itching and pain that go with hemorrhoids—the swollen veins in the anus and rectum that afflict many people over the age of 30. Drugstore shelves present the sufferer a confusing array of products compounded from 10 different types of drugs. Among these, none of the wound-healers, antiseptics, anticholinergics (nerve-impulse blockers) or miscellaneous ingredients—mostly traditional folk medicines—were recommended by the government reviewers.

Of the approved types some of the most widely used are the protectants—gels, creams, oils, lotions and the like that simply coat the affected area and physically protect it from irritation. Substances such as aluminum hydroxide gel, cocoa butter and shark-liver oil were among the many protectants approved, but the American Pharmaceutical Association said that ordinary petroleum jelly works just as well.

Among the other ingredients in hemorrhoid medicines, two pain-relievers—benzocaine and pramoxine hydrochloride—were found helpful. Three vasoconstrictors, drugs that cause temporary constriction of blood vessels, were approved—ephedrine sulfate, epinephrine hydrochloride, and phenylephrine hydrochloride. But these should be used with caution by those with diabetes, hyperthyroidism, high blood pressure and cardiovascular disease. Of available astringents, drugs applied to reduce inflammation, calamine, zinc oxide and witch hazel were recommended; menthol was approved as a counterirritant—a substance that distracts the sufferer from perceiving pain by creating a countervailing sensation—and alcloxa and resorcinol were approved as keratolytics, substances that reduce itching. All these substances come in many forms; ointments, creams, pastes and gels are considered equally useful. Some are made up in suppositories, but this form was held less useful by the American Pharmaceutical Association.

At last, skin remedies that work

Of all the nonprescription drugs, none have improved more radically than those intended for skin ailments—once among the most intractable of human afflictions. In the past, the work of the specialist in this field, the professional dermatologist, was wryly described as "the best specialty. The patient never dies—and never gets well." Today, getting well is a reasonable expectation.

That optimism stems from the efficacy of a number of new drugs now used to treat many of the old inflammations, itches and eruptions. Some skin ailments still resist cure. Baldness is one; the review panel found there was no product available that could prevent loss of hair or promote the growth of new hair. And the burn ointments on the market are more likely to harm than to help, irritating the wound or sealing the skin so that the heat cannot escape; cold water may be the best first aid for first-degree burns. But for sunburn, eczema, acne and dandruff there now are drugs that work.

Eczema—a catch-all name for sometimes maddening, sometimes painful inflammations and itches arising from various external causes—resisted even professional treatment until the 1950s. Then came the introduction of the prescription-only drugs called corticosteroids, which relieve symptoms but do not cure the illness causing the rash.

Most corticosteroids are potent and are capable of lowering resistance to infection, weakening the bones, inducing psychosis, causing hair to grow (though not on a bald head), bloating the face and abdomen, and even reactivating dormant tuberculosis. One corticosteroid, hydrocortisone, is an exception. After decades of professional use, a .5 per cent concentration was declared safe for external application without a doctor's supervision if not used for more than seven days. Almost overnight it became the home treatment for eczema and other irritations. Skin allergies or reactions to dry winter air, soaps, detergents, cosmetics, metal jewelry, poison ivy, poison oak, poison sumac and even insect bites became curable discomforts.

That scourge of teenagers, acne, has responded to creams or lotions containing benzoyl peroxide, available without prescription since 1976. In addition, the review panel found both sulfur and the combination sulfur-resorcinol effective agents. All act in the same way, peeling away inflamed skin cells so that they can be replaced by fresh ones. The American Pharmaceutical Association recommended beginning with the milder solutions of sulfur and sulfur-resorcinol before trying the more irritating benzoyl peroxide.

For dandruff—scales sloughed off when the scalp replaces its skin cells at an abnormally fast rate—successful treatment was found in shampoos that contain zinc pyrithione and selenium, introduced as a nonprescription 1 per cent solution in 1970. Both retard the production of new skin cells on the scalp. There are also milder remedies that contain sulfur, resorcinol or salicylic acid, which work by the opposite method, speeding the removal of scalp cells so that the scales do not accumulate.

The painful, potentially serious damage of sunburn is easy to avoid with clothing or by applying opaque ointments of zinc oxide or titanium dioxide to exposed skin. But even if there is no burn, exposure to the sun should be carefully controlled because it increases the risk of skin cancer. Such control is now provided by lotions termed sunscreens; one of the most commonly used types contains para-aminobenzoic acid, referred to as PABA.

Sunscreens are rated according to their sun protective factor, or SPF, which is displayed on most labels. The higher the SPF number, the longer the exposure to sunlight that can be tolerated without sunburn. A sunscreen rated SPF 4, for example, permits users to stay out in the sun four times as long without burning as they could if unprotected. How high an SPF rating is needed depends, of course, on the duration of exposure but also on the sensitivity of the individual's skin and on the intensity of the sun—the greatest protection is needed on the beach, on snowfields, on the water, in the tropics and at high altitudes.

Perhaps the most effective of the new drugs for skin ailments are two fungicides—compounds that eliminate the microscopic growths responsible for such ailments as ringworm, athlete's foot and jock itch. Several that have been on the market for years—undecylenic acid, calcium and zinc undecylenate, zinc stearate and benzoic acid, for example—were considered useful by the FDA antimicrobials panel. In 1971, however, a better compound, tolnaftate, was approved, and in 1980 the review panel recommended that a drug called miconazole be released for sale without a prescription. Miconazole works even faster than tolnaftate and is effective more often. It is one of the newer items in the growing list of nonprescription drugs that enable people to treat themselves for the most common ailments. ✳

HOW TO APPLY EYE MEDICINES
Clean secretions from the eyes with cotton. Then tilt your head back and toward the eye to be treated. Pull down the lower lid with one finger, forming a pouch (pink area). Looking up, squeeze the drops (left), or a quarter inch of ointment, into the pouch. Blink to distribute the medicine, then blot away any excess.

How to apply drops and ointments

If you have to administer eye, ear or nose medicines, the nurses' techniques illustrated on this page can help you get the greatest therapeutic effect out of the medicine. They can also help turn a possibly messy chore into a simple—and neat—operation. Regardless of which area you are medicating, you can minimize discomfort and potential contamination by following these common-sense rules.

First, wash your hands thoroughly. Draw the prescribed amount of medicine into the dropper, then administer the dose as shown in the drawings at right and below. Try not to let the applicator touch eyes, ears or nose—an admittedly difficult task, but one that helps prevent the spreading of infections. If you are using a dropper, return it to the bottle immediately; recap tubes equally promptly.

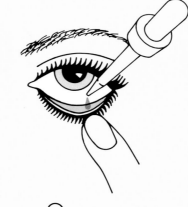

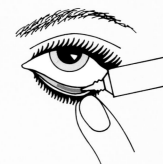

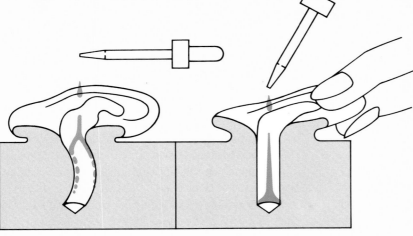

DO'S AND DON'TS OF USING EARDROPS
The natural curvature of the ear canal can prevent the medicine from reaching the eardrum (far left). To straighten the canal, lie on your side, exposing the ear to be treated, and gently pull the top of the ear upward and toward the back of your head (near left). Squeeze the dose into the canal. Remain on your side for about five minutes, then dry the ear.

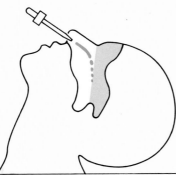

THE BEST WAY TO TAKE NOSE DROPS
Blow your nose gently, then sit upright and tilt your head back, using a pillow or other support if necessary. Push up on the tip of your nose to open the nasal passage, and insert the tip of the dropper about one third of an inch. Breathing through your mouth, administer the prescribed number of drops. Keep your head tilted back for a few moments to let the drops penetrate.

What the doctor orders

In the early part of this century, the entire arsenal of effective prescription drugs was small enough to fit into a doctor's black bag. Dr. Lewis Thomas, Chancellor of the Memorial Sloan-Kettering Cancer Center in New York City, described the drugs available to his father, a general practitioner who was graduated from medical school in 1904:

"In his doctor's bag that he carried off into the night on house calls was a handful of things. Morphine was the most important, and the only really indispensable drug in the whole pharmacopeia. Digitalis—for heart patients—was next in value. Insulin had arrived by the time he had been practicing for about 20 years, and he had it in his bag. Adrenalin was there in small glass ampoules in case he ran into a case of anaphylactic shock, which he never did."

The lifesaving cures taken for granted today did not exist. "There was nothing at all to do for someone stricken by acute rheumatic fever, or poliomyelitis, or meningitis, or tuberculosis." Nevertheless, he "wrote prescriptions of great complexity in Latin for almost all his patients," commented his son. "The pills were amulets warding off evil, and the prescriptions were incantations. If my father could have done a little dance at the bedside with his eyes rolled back, he would have qualified as a shaman in the ancient Indian tradition."

In the elder Thomas' time the practice of medicine consisted mainly of painstaking diagnosis of the patient's illness and thoughtful prediction of the outcome. The popular palliatives of the day had little biological effect, but when prescribed by a qualified physician in a sage, expert manner, they were often enough to comfort—and even cure—many patients.

When, decades later, powerfully effective drugs became available, the cures they brought seemed like miracles. "Early in my medical career," Dr. Robert S. Mendelsohn of Chicago remembered, "I gave intravenous penicillin every few hours to children who were suffering the agonizing symptoms of bacterial meningitis, and then watched miraculous changes occur hour by hour. Children who had been on the verge of death recovered consciousness and began to respond to stimuli within a few hours. A few days later those same children were back on their feet, almost ready to go home. Patients with lobar pneumonia also would endure terrible agonies. Some recovered, but many died. When penicillin came along, people with lobar pneumonia no longer went through a crisis period."

The magical power of prescription drugs still works and is used by every good physician. But today's drugs cure not only by magic but also by direct action on disease. Some 1,500 potent chemicals—in about 41,000 prescription drug products, the most effective of them developed since World War II—are now at the doctor's disposal. And American doctors prescribe them in staggering numbers. Some 1.4 billion prescriptions, or about seven for every man, woman and child in the United States, are filled by drugstores each year. Millions more are filled in hospitals and public clinics.

The explosion of new and powerful drugs has saved the lives of millions of people and has eased pain and discomfort for millions more. It has also cost lives and pain. Modern

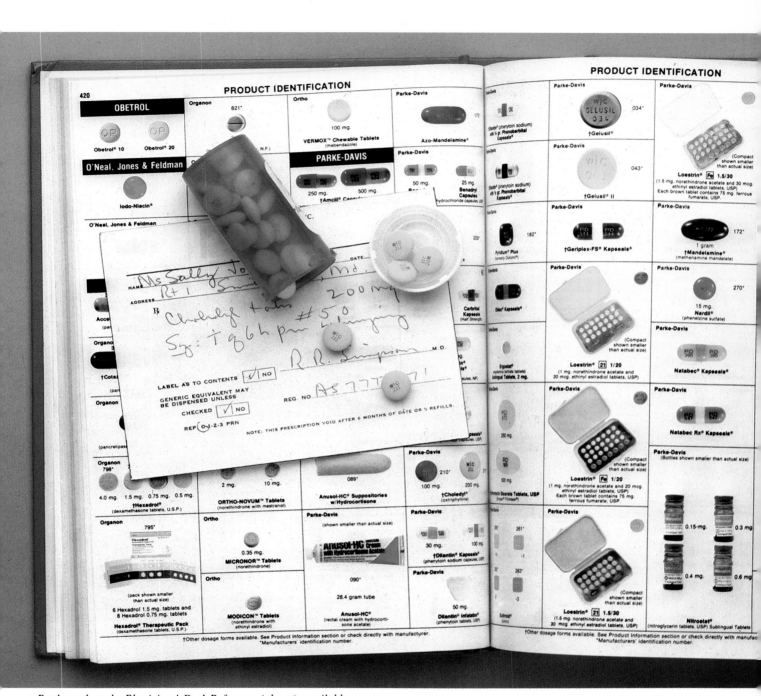

Books such as the Physicians' Desk Reference (above), available for customers' use in many pharmacies, make it easy to check on prescriptions and labels. Simply look up the name of the medicine prescribed—here, the antiasthmatic Choledyl —then compare the product with the drug's picture (center, third from bottom). Shape, color and identifying marks should match.

prescription drugs are so diverse and prescribing them is so complex that the chance for error is alarming. Everyone has stories about incorrect prescriptions—the ulcer patient given a cold remedy containing ulcer-exacerbating aspirin, the person allergic to penicillin who died soon after an injection. The huge number of prescriptions is only one sign that many more drugs are taken than are needed. But even the most carefully considered prescription entails some risk, and neither doctor nor patient can be certain of the result. "When a patient takes any prescription drug for the first time, he or she is in fact participating in an experiment under the physician's direction," said Dr. James Long, Health Services Director for the National Science Foundation.

One reason for the experimental nature of prescribing is the potency of prescription drugs, which are as a rule stronger than those available over the counter. As much knowledge and judgment are required to prescribe such drugs correctly as to make the correct diagnosis in the first place. Once the doctor decides that a medicine is needed, he must then determine which one, in what strength, at what dosage and for how long. Because the drug works by interacting with body chemistry, the physician must consider the patient's sex, age, weight, medical history, ancestry, eating and drinking habits and other medicines the patient may be taking—in addition to the illness being treated. These are only some of the factors that may influence the effects of a drug.

Dr. William A. Nolen, author of *The Making of a Surgeon,* drew from his experience with a common tranquilizer a sample of the unpredictable variety in drug effects a doctor might meet: "One of my patients, a forty-five-year-old man who weighs one hundred ninety pounds and is six feet tall, practically falls asleep if he takes two and a half milligrams of Valium. His wife, who is thirty-five years old, stands five feet six inches tall and weighs one hundred twenty-five pounds, requires ten milligrams for even mild sedation. Apparently, either their bodies metabolize Valium at different rates or their brain cells differ in susceptibility to the drug."

With so many influences at work, the patient must share responsibility with the physician for the drug experiments entailed in treatment. The patient must make sure the doctor understands everything about his life and habits that may affect results. Almost anything can exert some influence. For example, nicotine can speed up the way the body uses and eliminates pentazocine, a painkiller, and smokers may need more of the drug to reduce pain than nonsmokers. Drugs used to treat diseases of the veins and arteries can induce a tendency to hypothermia—a deep drop in body temperature—which can be fatal if not treated promptly.

Not all physicians take the proper precautions. In one instance, when a frail elderly woman's blood pressure dropped drastically at the start of surgery for a broken hip, a review of preoperative prescriptions showed that she had received a standard dose of Demerol instead of a dose reduced to fit her age and weight. The surgery was postponed.

The patient must be made to understand all the unintended side effects a drug might have as well as all the effects it is intended to have. He must take his medicines as instructed; a surprising number of people do not. He must be alert for unexpected reactions. The standard advice of the experts is: If a medicine makes you sick instead of better, check with your doctor before taking any more.

The physician's role in this dual responsibility demands ongoing technical education in the characteristics of drugs and close attention to professional reports. The patient's role demands some knowledge of what the doctor knows—and of how that information was obtained.

The ills prescription drugs cure

Of all the drugs a doctor prescribes, most are likely to come from among only 10 types, classified according to the disorder or discomfort they alleviate.

The most-prescribed drugs are:
● Anti-infectives. Beginning with sulfa drugs in 1936 and the original antibiotic, penicillin, in the 1940s, these medicines were the first of a generation of powerful new drugs. Such compounds as tetracycline, erythromycin and a whole family of penicillin variants are produced by many companies and are among the most commonly prescribed drugs. Antibiotics now exist to combat virtually every bacterial infection that afflicts humans. Antibiotics kill the target bacte-

ria by disrupting their normal growth or life processes *(page 82)*. They are of no help in viral infections.

● Drugs for high blood pressure. Diuretics reduce blood pressure by increasing urine production to lessen the volume of fluid in the blood. Hydralazine (Apresoline) acts directly on blood-vessel walls to relax them. So-called beta blockers such as propranolol (Inderal) block the actions of nerves that constrict the blood vessels, while methyldopa (Aldomet) decreases the activity of nerve centers in the brain, thereby reducing the ability of nerves to constrict blood vessels.

● Pain-relieving, or analgesic, medicines. The leading brands are combinations of over-the-counter painkillers—aspirin or acetaminophen—and some type of stronger but potentially habit-forming painkilling compound, generally codeine. A narcotic, codeine is derived from opium and, like the more effective but far more addictive morphine, it binds to receptors in the central nervous system to relieve pain. In use since 1886, codeine yields few serious side effects or adverse reactions and carries almost no risk of addiction if used in moderate doses for short times. Aspirin with codeine reduces both inflammation and pain caused by rheumatism or arthritis. Acetaminophen has no anti-inflammatory powers but taken with codeine is an excellent analgesic.

● Heart-disease drugs. The beta blockers not only control blood pressure but also reduce heart pain by interfering with nerve actions, thereby slowing heartbeat and lowering blood pressure. Beta blockers are now replacing the older heart medicines such as digitalis, nitroglycerin and quinidine.

● Allergy drugs. Most are either antihistamines, such as chlorpheniramine (Chlor-Trimeton), which block the typical inflaming action of histamine; or combinations of antihistamines with phenylpropanolamine—decongestant drugs that constrict blood vessels, allowing obstructed breathing passages to open up. These prescription drugs are more powerful than formulations available over the counter.

● Arthritis medicines. Several prescription drugs, including ibuprofen (Motrin), naproxen (Naprosyn) and fenoprofen calcium (Nalfon), have much the same effects as aspirin—reduction of pain, inflammation and fever—but generally cause less stomach upset than do the large doses of

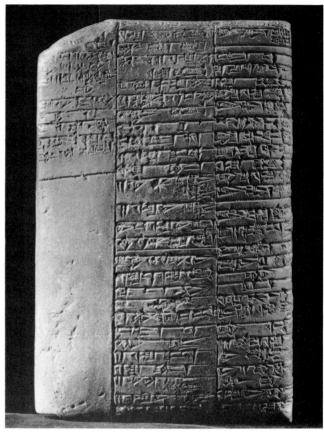

A 4,000-year-old clay tablet from Sumeria is inscribed in cuneiform writing with history's earliest known medical prescriptions. One prescription consists of ground tortoise shell, salt, mustard and beer. But the tablet does not reveal the ailments that its medicines were meant to cure.

aspirin needed by people severely stricken by arthritis.
● Minor tranquilizers (so called to distinguish them from the ones used only for the severely disturbed). Meprobamate (Miltown), Chlordiazepoxide (Librium) and diazepam (Valium) all give short-term relief from mild anxiety. Some five billion tranquilizer pills are prescribed annually, with about 33 million prescriptions written for Valium alone.
● Sleeping aids. Flurazepam (Dalmane) is the most popular relief for insomnia. Its method of action is still not known.
● Oral contraceptives. These estrogenic and progestational hormones, which prevent the production and release of egg cells, are used by more than seven million American women.
● Ulcer drugs. Few medicines were much better for this common ailment than nonprescription antacids until the introduction in 1977 of cimetidine *(Chapter 6),* which quickly became the ulcer medicine most prescribed by physicians.

These 10 types of drugs are the ones most prescribed, simply because they generally work. Yet also widely used are a great many prescription remedies whose effectiveness is in doubt. Since 1962 the makers of any prescription drug have had to prove with two or more scientific studies that their medicine works substantially as they claim, before they

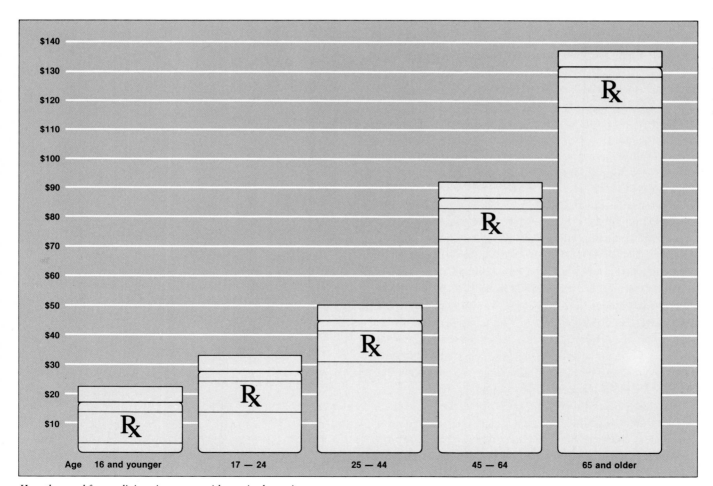

How the need for medicines increases with age is shown in this graph of the annual per capita expenditures for prescriptions of five age groups. The elderly use more prescriptions—an average of 18 per year compared to four for the youngest group— and pay more for each one. And at any age, females use more medicines than males, and the poor more than those better off.

can receive a license to sell it in the United States. At the time this legal requirement took effect, some 3,500 prescription drugs were on the market. The Food and Drug Administration (FDA), along with the National Academy of Sciences and its National Research Council, reviewed this pharmacopeia and divided the drugs into 30 different categories, such as antibiotics, antihistamines, analgesics, vasodilators, cardiorenal and metabolic drugs. A panel for each drug group was formed, made up of six experts who analyzed the drugs' effectiveness. These panels determined that for at least 450 prescription drugs, effectiveness had not been proved.

In some cases, even after manufacturers' claims have been proved to be unsubstantiated, the attempt to remove a drug from the marketplace has led to a battle that has seemed endless. Trexinest, which combines lututrin—a hormone from sows' ovaries—with an estrogen and is prescribed for menopausal problems, was removed from the list of accepted drugs without any protest from the manufacturer. However, when the FDA Commissioner proposed that lututrin, which was prescribed as Lutrexin for menstrual cramps, premature labor and threatened miscarriages, also be removed, the manufacturer filed a complaint before the U.S. District Court, questioning the FDA's action on both Lutrexi and Trexinest. After seven years of court battles that went as far as the Supreme Court, both drugs were taken off the FDA's list of approved drugs because the manufacturer had failed to prove that the active ingredient, lututrin, was effective. Until that time, both drugs were still sold to the public.

Unproved drugs must be so labeled until the FDA can make a final evaluation. The notice describes the conditions or diseases for which the drug was found to be ''probably effective,'' ''possibly effective,'' or ''lacking substantial evidence of effectiveness.'' Yet doctors still prescribe them: One out of every eight prescriptions, about a billion dollars' worth a year, is for such a questionable medicine.

When a prescription is not best

The lack of experimental proof of biological effect does not necessarily mean that a drug will not work. Subtle biological actions are often missed in drug trials. And almost anything, if administered with confident authority, will make some people feel better—sometimes. Shamans achieve astonishingly high cure rates with dances and chicken sacrifices.

A patient making a costly visit to the doctor expects, if not a ceremonial dance, at least more than just advice. Said Jere E. Goyan, former commissioner of the FDA, ''Many patients have come to think that their visit to the doctor is not complete or worthwhile unless they walk away with a prescription. So consumer expectations for drugs are high.'' The result is the prescription not only of questionable drugs but also of too many drugs of unquestionable potency. Some time during the first two centuries of the Roman Empire, according to the medical historian Elinore Peebles, one citizen of Rome remarked that the average person, when sick, ''promptly visited his doctor, for he realized that doctors must live, then obediently filled his prescription, for of course, the druggist had to live; after which he took the medicine home and threw it out of the window because he himself had to live.''

Overprescribing often makes tragic headlines. After entertainer Elvis Presley was found dead in his Memphis mansion in 1977, the state Board of Medical Examiners investigated. Its 59-page complaint charged that the singer had been given some 12,000 pills and vials of drugs—tranquilizers, stimulants, sedatives, painkillers—in the last 18 months of his life. The license of his physician was suspended.

Such disasters are fortunately rare, but overprescribing is not. A study of thousands of outpatient prescriptions, conducted by the Los Angeles County-University of Southern California Medical Center, revealed that an unacceptably high percentage involved excessive amounts, repeated prescriptions for the same drug or inappropriate concurrent prescriptions for different drugs.

One outpatient, it was discovered, had been given a total of 54 prescriptions in less than four months, including 12 on a single day. During the four-month period he received, among other drugs: 870 capsules of a minor tranquilizer and 40 tablets of a major one; 1,130 capsules of a painkiller, plus 200 aspirin tablets and 300 of an aspirin substitute; 520 tablets of one kind of arthritic drug and 240 of another; 700

capsules of an anticonvulsant, 500 tablets of nitroglycerin for heart pains and 530 tablets of two medicines for high blood pressure; 500 tablets of a barbiturate; 620 capsules of an antibiotic and 40 of an anti-infective; 300 thyroid tablets and 300 tablets of multiple vitamins. Miraculously, he lived.

Obviously, doctors who prescribe so indiscriminately are to be avoided. "The first rule of therapy," noted Dr. W. T. Thompson, editor of *Virginia Medical,* "is 'First do not harm.' And sometimes akin to it is the admonition: 'Don't just do something; stand there.' " But even the wisest physician needs the patient's cooperation in avoiding unnecessary use of medicines. There are many responses to illness, and taking drugs is only one of them. In every case, both patient and physician must weigh benefits and risks and decide whether to use medicines, to try an alternative therapy or to adopt Dr. Thompson's suggestion and simply stand there.

A muscle strain, for example, might seem to demand a painkiller. But many such drugs cause drowsiness; if the victim drives a car, runs heavy machinery or has a job requiring special alertness, the wisest course may be to pass up a drug and choose instead bandaging, rest and ice periodically for a day or two. On the other hand, a seemingly minor problem may require strong medicine to prevent serious complications. Children's earaches, for example, are so common and usually so brief that many are treated casually. But if the infection causing an earache is not soon eliminated with antibiotics, it can lead to meningitis or hearing loss.

How the physician knows

A sound decision on the use of prescriptions must depend largely on a doctor's understanding of drug action—yet the depth of this understanding is, in the opinion of many authorities, quite variable. Because developments in pharmacology have come so rapidly since World War II, keeping up is difficult. And because these developments are so widely reported in the news, some patients find themselves in the uncomfortable position of knowing about a drug or a drug reaction that their physicians have never heard of.

Doctors learn about the drugs they prescribe from several sources, including their own study at medical school, promotional information from drug companies, reference works, professional journals and newsletters, and hospital drug-information centers.

Formal schooling may be the least of these sources, although it is basic. The foundation of a doctor's knowledge of drugs is typically laid during the second of the four years at medical school, in 60 to 120 class hours of review of all drug types. Most students learn more about medicines and prescribing from comments of professors or visiting superstars of medicine—statements that, however offhand, may have deeper effect than a second-year course in basic science. Explained Dr. Richard Burack in his *New Handbook of Prescription Drugs:* "Students cease to learn in depth about drugs, and while they continue to receive first-rate instruction in pathological physiology, diagnosis, and surgical treatment, they begin to adopt sloppy prescribing habits."

To reinforce the future doctor's drug knowledge, most universities offer more pharmacology courses in the last two years of medical school—the clinical years spent working with patients in hospitals. For practicing physicians, medical schools also offer continuing-education courses in pharmacology, but these are not widespread nor much attended.

By far the most influential source of information on new medicines is the drug companies. They spend more than one billion dollars a year to promote prescription drugs to physicians—about $3,000 for every doctor in the United States. Much of that promotional work is carried out by "detail men"—so called because they are trained to provide detailed information on various drug products. Some 20,000 of these sales representatives call on doctors throughout the country. Surveys have shown that doctors obtain a third to a half of their knowledge of new drugs from detail men.

These are no ordinary salesmen. Most are college graduates, and many have degrees in health or in such biological sciences as biochemistry and genetics. More than three quarters of the Eli Lilly Company's 1,000 or so sales representatives, for example, are pharmacists.

Perhaps what most sets the detail man apart from other sales people is that he sells the idea of a product, rather than the product itself, to the doctor. This has significant implications for the patient, a person the detail man never sees or talks to, but the one who pays for the product.

As someone who learns about the product but who never needs to buy it, the doctor often does not investigate the cost of a drug. A 1973 FDA survey of 10,000 physicians showed that 30 per cent never try to find out how much their prescriptions cost. When they do seek price information, they generally ask the detail man rather than a pharmacist, who could give actual store prices of competitive products.

The detail man's wish to show his goods in the best light could lead to excesses of zeal in touting drugs' powers and minimizing their drawbacks. But all drug promotion, whether detail men's efforts or advertising in professional journals, is carefully regulated by two complementary watchdog agencies. The FDA's Division of Drug Advertising and Labeling reviews all advertising materials, including promotion for prescription drugs, and can compel manufacturers to circulate retractions of inaccurate or misleading information.

The drug industry, through the Pharmaceutical Manufacturers Association, also polices itself. Its Code of Fair Practices in the Promotion of Drug Products lays down standards of accuracy and clarity, correct quotation of medical authorities, and fair comparison of drugs. Balancing in some ways the influence of the detail men is the mass of printed material available to physicians. Many of the journals—there are more than 8,000 medical periodicals published by professional societies such as the American Medical Association and the American College of Surgeons, and by commercial enterprises—provide technical articles on drugs. Almost all journals also are heavy with drug advertisements, which are based upon information that has been reviewed by the FDA.

Looking it up—the reference books

The journals provide background, but for everyday use in prescribing for patients, a doctor is most likely to turn to one of several reference books. *The Merck Manual* gives brief descriptions of ailments and the standard treatments for them. The United States Pharmacopeial Convention's *USP Dispensing Information* is a compendium of information on most drugs approved for use in the United States, as is *AMA*

Drug Evaluations, which also includes selected Canadian products. But the most widely used source of specifics on drugs is the *Physicians' Desk Reference,* or *PDR,* which is distributed to all practicing American doctors, free of charge, in a new edition each year. A Congressional survey of 10,000 doctors in 1973 found that they used this 2,000-page, two-inch-thick volume an average of 7.5 times per week.

The *PDR* is primarily an advertising vehicle. The extensive information given is written by the manufacturer, who pays to have it included. The information is the standard, government-approved data that appears in advertisements in medical journals and in the package inserts that accompany shipments of the drug to the pharmacist or doctor.

Although these references use technical language, understanding them does not require a medical degree. All of the books are available in most public libraries and many drugstores, and a good deal of directly useful information can be gleaned from them. Of the three, the *PDR* is the most popular source of drug data for patients as well as for physicians. A section from it is reproduced in the illustration on page 53.

The *PDR* lists drugs by maker and, under each company's name, by the brand names of its products. Information on the arthritis medicine sulindac, for example, appears under the name of its manufacturer, Merck Sharpe & Dohme, and under its brand name, Clinoril. The drug's generic name and its chemical composition and type are given first. Next is a section called "clinical pharmacology," listing the drug's therapeutic effects: sulindac is an "anti-inflammatory drug, also possessing analgesic and antipyretic activities," i.e., it relieves swelling, pain and fever. Then come brief reports on studies of the drug's effectiveness in several kinds of arthritis, bursitis and spinal inflammation.

The key information for the prescribing doctor and the patient alike comes next in sulindac's two-page entry. First are its "indications," a simple listing of the specific ailments for which it is approved—those that were discussed at length in the pharmacology section.

Next comes an entire page of admonitory information under no less than five different headings: "Contraindications" are cases in which the drug should not be used—such as for

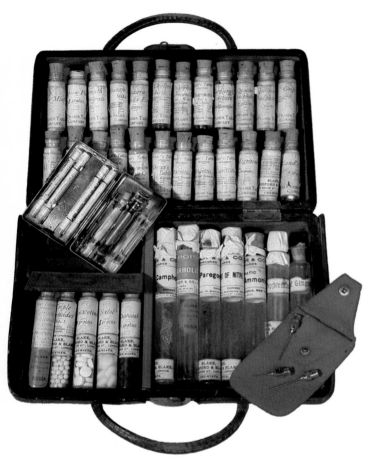

A portable medicine kit—such as this one, carried throughout Asia and Europe in the early 20th Century by American diplomat Irwin Laughlin—was until recently a practical necessity for prudent travelers. Few kits were as elaborate as Laughlin's, which included a hypodermic, a cocaine drug for voice loss, and corrosive sublimate, a powerful antiseptic for flesh wounds.

"patients who are hypersensitive to this product" and for those who react allergically to aspirin. "Warnings" tell of the dangers of ulcers and gastrointestinal bleeding. Under the "Precautions" heading comes a general statement followed by subsections on "use in pregnancy," "nursing mothers," "use in children" and "drug interactions."

"Adverse reactions" are also subdivided—into those that occurred in more than 1 per cent of the 1,865 patients who took sulindac in clinical tests, those seen in less than 1 per cent and those that occurred so rarely they could not be clearly blamed on the drug. Finally, under "management of overdosage" are emergency instructions to counter misuse.

Following this catalogue of admonitions, the section on "dosage and administration" contains the information the doctor will use in writing instructions on the prescription—how to take the medicine, how much, how often. Different dosages are recommended for different ailments.

The last item, "how supplied," tells whether the drug is available in tablets, capsules, liquid, salves or other forms, and gives the color of the pill or package. A separate section in the *PDR,* of special value to the patient, contains full-color photographs of most medicines, many of them actual size. Because each capsule or tablet has a unique appearance—shape, color and markings—a patient can usually check the drug sold by a pharmacist against its picture to make sure the medicine he gets is the one prescribed.

In 1962, the first of a new kind of information source appeared—the drug-information center. Serving doctors and patients who wish to find out about a specific drug or how to treat a specific illness, such centers have become increasingly important; 86 had been established by early 1976.

Drug-information centers fit no single description. Most are connected with the department of pharmacology of a hospital or medical center. Some, like the one at the Brookdale Hospital Medical Center in Brooklyn, New York, serve mainly the hospital's doctors and nurses. Others, such as the center at the Arnold and Marie Schwartz College of Pharmacy and Health Sciences, Long Island University, serve physicians, nurses, pharmacists and the drug industry itself. "We are asked the type of questions not readily found in conven-

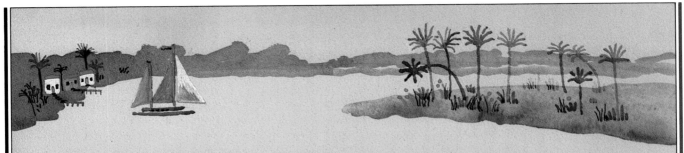

The shots a traveler needs

A trip outside the supposedly sanitary United States once required not only a personal kit of home-bought medicines *(opposite)* but an official document, the International Certificates of Vaccination, attesting to vaccinations against several diseases. Today most communicable diseases are under control in most places, and the only immunization visitors need is the one for yellow fever, stipulated by some countries in Africa and South America. However, tourists planning to venture beyond modern cities may also need preventives for diseases that are still a hazard where unsanitary conditions prevail. Immunizations recommended by the Centers for Disease Control are listed below. In addition, protection against tetanus (lockjaw) is important at home as well as abroad.

It still is wise to take along a supply of any medicines routinely used, as well as a diarrhea cure for that travelers' complaint. Pharmacists abroad may not honor prescriptions written in the United States, and over-the-counter brands and sizes are unfamiliar—the aspirin pills commonly used in France contain almost twice as much aspirin as the ordinary American tablets.

DISEASE	AREAS OF PREVALENCE	PREVENTIVE	DURATION OF PROTECTION
MALARIA	Parts of Asia, Africa, the Middle East, Central and South America, Haiti and New Guinea	Oral drug, chloroquine, taken once a week beginning 7 days before arrival in the area and continuing 6 weeks after leaving. An additional drug combination, pyrimethamine and sulfadoxine, is needed upon arrival in some areas.	Effective only while pills are being taken
MEASLES	Worldwide	Single vaccine injection 2 weeks before departure, needed only by people who have never had the disease or the vaccination	Lifetime
POLIO	Tropical or developing countries	For unvaccinated adults, 4 doses of the injected vaccine (IPV) over 12 months; for unvaccinated children, 3 doses of the oral vaccine (OPV) over 12 months	5 to 10 years for IPV, after which a booster dose is needed; lifetime for OPV
TETANUS-DIPHTHERIA	Worldwide	3 vaccine injections over 12 months	10 years, after which a booster injection is needed
TYPHOID FEVER	Sections of Africa, Asia, Central and South America	2 vaccine injections 4 weeks apart	3 years, after which a booster dose is needed
VIRAL HEPATITIS, TYPE A	Sections of tropical or developing countries	Single gamma globulin injection about 24 hours before departure	3 to 5 months, after which a repeat injection is needed
YELLOW FEVER	Parts of Africa, South America	Single vaccine injection at least 10 days before departure	10 years, after which vaccination must be repeated

How to read a prescription

The immediate result of most visits to the doctor is a prescription, cryptic but usually readable with the help of a glossary of the common abbreviations *(below)*.

Although Latin abbreviations sometimes serve as a shorthand, English is used more often. And most prescriptions contain the same information: the date, the doctor's and patient's name and address; the name, form, strength and quantity of the drug; instructions for use; and how many times the prescription may be refilled. As for the familiar Rx that has come to mean ''prescription''—it may come from either the Latin word *recipe,* meaning ''you take,'' or the classical symbol for the god Jupiter, who was traditionally invoked in prayer on prescriptions.

aa. of each	**pil.** pill
a.c. before meals	**p.o.** by mouth
ad lib. as often as desired	**p.r.n.** as needed
alt. hor. every other hour	**pulv.** powder
b.i.d. twice daily	**q.** every
c. with	**q. 4 h.** every four hours
caps. capsule	**q.d.** every day
et and	**q.h.** every hour
fl. or fld. fluid	**q.i.d.** four times a day
g or gm. gram (.03333 ounce)	**q.s.** as much as required
gr. grain (.00228 ounce)	**s.** without
gtt. drop (.00166 fluid ounce)	**sig.** write, mark or label
h. hour	**sol.** solution
h.s. at bedtime	**ss.** half
mg. milligram (.00003 ounce)	**stat.** immediately
non r. not to be repeated	**tab.** tablet
o.d. right eye	**t.i.d.** three times a day
o.s. left eye	**tr.** tincture
o.u. both eyes	**ung.** ointment
p.c. after meals	**ut. dict.** as directed

tional resources—not the sort you can go to the *PDR* for,'' said its assistant director, Harold Kirschenbaum.

The Consumer's Drug Information Service at the St. Francis Medical Center in Lynwood, California, is oriented toward patients. It responds to more than 300 telephone inquiries a month, more than half about prescription drugs. The most frequent questions were about side-effects and adverse reactions, drug identification and therapeutic uses.

How to help the doctor choose the drug

A well-informed doctor and patient should be able to cooperate in a prudent use of medicines. That they often do not is blamed by many experts on lack of communication in the doctor's office. ''The real villain of the piece,'' observed a physician who studied the pattern in several thousand government employees, ''is the 10-minute interview, which in some cases is only six or eight. Under the time pressures of medical practice today, it takes a wise and efficient doctor indeed—not to mention a wise and attentive patient—to exchange enough vital information in the brief time of the average office visit to ensure not only that the right treatment is prescribed but that it is understood and carried out.''

Several strategies help make the most of a physician's time and talent, to ensure that you not only get the right medicine but get the most out of it. The first is so basic that it is sometimes overlooked: Get the facts straight in advance of the visit. Write down all the information you have and take it with you to the doctor's office. Start with the symptoms you have experienced, when and how often they occurred, and how long they lasted; note anything that seems to make the symptoms diminish or increase.

Equally crucial is your medical history. Be prepared to tell the doctor of any long-term illnesses in your family: There may be hereditary factors in such diseases as diabetes and hypertension. List your own past illnesses, medicines taken for them and the effectiveness of the treatment.

Be sure to include all current health conditions you may have and what drugs you are taking for them; whether prescription or over-the-counter. If you are not sure of the exact name or nature of a drug, bring the labeled bottle with you.

This is information your doctor must have to avoid prescribing a new medicine that will interact dangerously with what you are already taking.

Do not forget that over-the-counter medicines are also drugs, and that when used together with prescription medicines they can produce unwanted and even serious effects. Almost every doctor has heard a patient exclaim, "Oh, I didn't know aspirin was a drug!"

Certain foods and beverages, too, can react with drugs. Tetracycline is a common example: It should not be taken with dairy products, whose calcium content interferes with its absorption.

Let the doctor know about any adverse reaction or unpleasant side effects you have experienced with any drug in the past. Antibiotics, particularly the widely used penicillins, account for a high percentage of allergic reactions. If you are allergic to penicillin, moreover, you will probably be allergic to other drugs in the same group, such as ampicillin.

Giving the doctor all the pertinent information is only half the job. You also have to make sure the doctor tells you everything you need to know. You have a legal right and a responsibility to yourself to ask precisely what the diagnosis is and to discuss the proposed course of treatment.

It takes diplomacy to bring up alternatives—medicines you have heard about, generic substitutes or possible non-drug treatments. One physician commented, "If a patient comes in with notes, an M.D. may say to himself, 'Oh, here comes another one of *those* guys.' " And although you are a partner in your treatment, your doctor is still the expert.

Once a drug is prescribed, make sure you know its name; if necessary, have the doctor carefully pronounce it and spell it out for you. Many very different drugs have brand names or generic names so similar that there is real danger of confusion. Orinase is an antidiabetic drug; Ornade a decongestant. Ask the doctor to show you a color picture of the drug in the *PDR* or some other reference source, or to show you a sample of it, so you know what it looks like and will be able to check it when you fill the prescription.

The doctor should tell you exactly what to expect from the drug: how it should affect your illness, how soon you should see signs of change and what side effects may arise.

Ask the doctor to read the prescription to you in detail. Ideally, you should receive a set of written instructions for taking the drug; if you do not, make notes of what the doctor tells you. The information should include how many times a day the drug is to be taken and at what intervals. Get explicit instructions: If told to take a pill "three times a day," ask if that means morning, noon and night, or at precise eight-hour intervals. Should a drug to be taken at mealtimes be swallowed before, during or after the meal? How long should you continue to take the drug?

It is even wise in some cases to ask how to take the drug. *The New England Journal of Medicine* reported the case of a hospital patient whose doctor gave him a container of liquid antiseptic soap with which to shower before surgery. But the doctor did not specify what to do with it. The patient drank the soap and eventually complained to the doctor that the medicine he had been given made him vomit. That is an extreme case, to be sure, but most doctors regale their friends with similar stories, all caused by a lack of communication.

All these instructions should be included in the prescription the doctor gives you. You are likely to have trouble reading it, and not only because physicians' handwriting is notoriously illegible. For centuries physicians wrote their prescriptions entirely in Latin, partly to create an aura of mystery and keep the patient in the dark, but also for the practical reason that Latin was the universal language of science, with precise meanings an apothecary could interpret when mixing a potion. Today vestiges of the Latin tradition persist, despite the urgings of medical associations that doctors write prescriptions in common language. Most of these cryptic notations are abbreviations that are well known to physicians and pharmacists and save doctors time. With some effort and a glossary of abbreviations *(opposite)* you can decode prescriptions, but it is more important that you make sure your pharmacist translates them fully and accurately into clear language when typing the label.

The label should include several kinds of information. Most important are the drug name and instructions for use. Traditionally, the name of the drug was omitted from the

Ingenious aids for taking medicine

For a medicine to work, it must be taken—and at the right time and in the right amount. Yet one study reported that as many as one third of all patients regularly fail to follow their physicians' instructions for taking medicines. Such noncompliance is often unintentional. Some people find it difficult to remember exactly when they took their last pills. Others have trouble swallowing a pill or an unpleasant-tasting liquid without gagging and coughing it up. Still others unwittingly use inaccurate measuring devices—the teaspoon specified on a medicine label is meant to contain one sixth of an ounce, but household teaspoons, including those used to measure baking ingredients, can vary from less than half to twice that capacity.

To help patients follow their physicians' orders, a number of drugstores now offer a variety of simple gadgets such as those in the representative sampling pictured on these pages. Memory aids *(below)* that help organize and monitor pill-taking on a daily and weekly basis are especially useful if several different drugs must be consumed daily, or if pills must be taken on a complex schedule. Specially designed plastic drinking glasses *(right, top)* make pill-swallowing easier and more convenient. And carefully calibrated syringes, droppers and spoons *(right, bottom)* ensure accurate measuring. Most measures are marked in teaspoons as well as in the metric system's cubic centimeters (cc.) or milliliters (ml.), which are identical units equivalent to $1/30$ ounce.

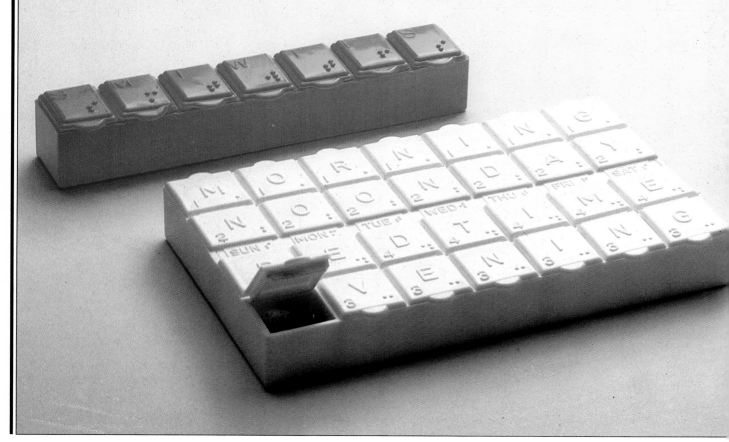

PILL ORGANIZERS
Dispensers with compartments for each day of the week help patients keep track of the medicines they have taken. These dispensers hold from one (top) to four (bottom) daily doses. Raised letters and Braille symbols indicate the day (top) or the day and time of day (bottom) that the pills should be taken.

PILL-DISPENSING GLASS
A special plastic tumbler helps people swallow pills. The glass is partly filled with water, then a pill is placed inside on the fluted shelf. When the tumbler is tipped, pill and water flow out together.

TRAVELING PILL CASE AND CUP
This collapsible plastic cup—like the ones children take to summer camp—has a storage compartment in its lid for pills. With the cup-and-pill assembly, a pill can be taken wherever drinking water is available.

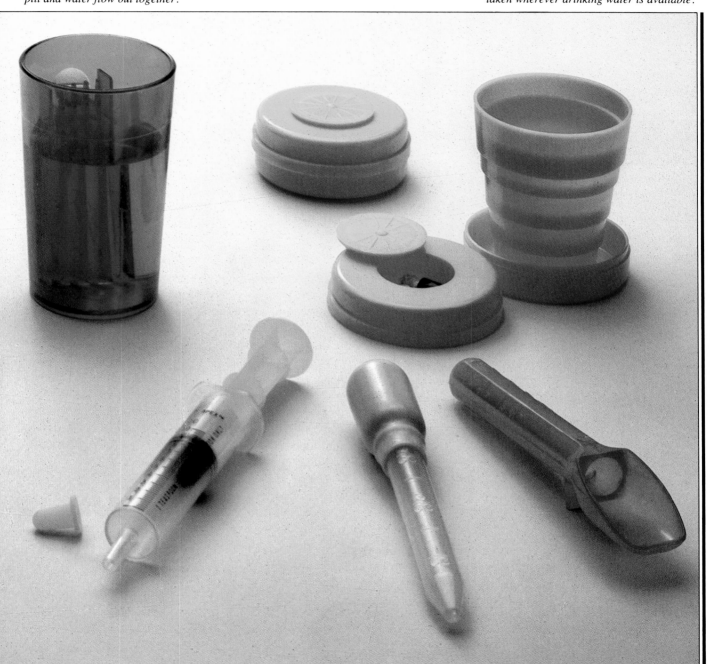

ORAL SYRINGE
The oral syringe makes it easy to squirt accurately measured doses of liquid medicines—up to two teaspoons—directly into the mouth of a young child. The tip is designed so it cannot hold a needle.

ORAL MEDICINE DROPPER
Like the oral syringe at left, the dropper above can be used to dispense medicine at the back of the mouth—beyond the taste buds—to help prevent gagging. The dropper holds a full teaspoon.

MEDICINE SPOON
Inscribed on the hollow handle of a plastic spoon are precise markings that measure up to 10 cc., or two full teaspoons, of liquid medicine. A leg lets the spoon rest on a flat surface without spilling its contents.

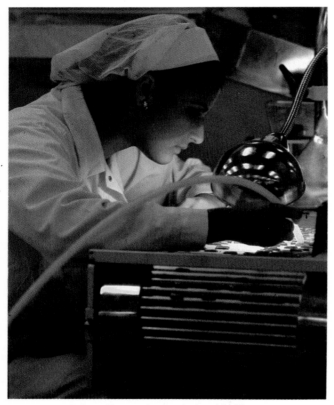

Using a simple but effective device—a hand-held vacuum hose—an inspector in a pharmaceutical plant sucks out defective antibiotic capsules as they pass her checkpoint on a slow-moving conveyor. Broken, chipped or incompletely filled capsules shuttle through the vacuum hose to a reject bin; the pills that pass inspection drop from the conveyor and later are packaged.

label, but today most doctors instruct the pharmacist to give it—by noting on the prescription slip "Label as such," "L.A.S." or simply "Label"—unless in rare circumstances they are concerned that the information may cause the patient psychological damage. The drug name is essential: Not only does it prevent mix-ups and provide an immediate record of medication if a patient changes doctors or moves to a new town, but it can prove a lifesaving means of identification in an emergency.

It is unwise to accept a prescription slip that ends with the notation "Ut dict." or "UD"—or its English equivalent, "as directed." Even if you understood those directions in the doctor's office, a few days later you may be hazy on them or may confuse them with the directions for another drug.

Getting the right dose at the right time

Once you have a prescription and the necessary instructions, all that remains to be done is to fill the prescription promptly at a pharmacy and take the drugs as directed—in medical parlance, to comply with the treatment.

Elementary as this may sound, a startlingly large number of patients fail to comply with their doctor's orders. Hippocrates, almost 2,400 years ago, warned doctors to "keep a watch also on the faults of the patients, which often make them lie about the taking of things prescribed. For through not taking disagreeable drinks, purgatives or other, they sometimes die. What they have done never results in a confession, but the blame is thrown upon the physician."

The problem has not gone away. In a 1979 survey by the Upjohn Company of 1,006 men and women of above-average education and income, 35 per cent admitted that at one time or another they had obtained a prescription from a doctor and not had it filled at all; the major reason, given by 62 per cent, was that the medicine was "not needed" (cost was cited by only 12 per cent). Some 70 per cent had failed to take all the medicine in a prescription they had filled, either because they felt they had "recovered from the condition" (59 per cent), "didn't need it" (25 per cent) or had experienced unpleasant side effects (10 per cent). None of these explanations is a valid reason for stopping a course of treatment without consulting the doctor. Prescribed medicines continue to do their work even after symptoms are no longer perceived, and though side effects should be reported to the physician, they are not in themselves an adequate cause for abandoning a medicine without his approval.

In another study, only 48 per cent of adult diabetics giving themselves insulin were actually found to be administering the prescribed dose. Research in a private practice in Rochester, New York, showed that only 55 per cent of patients told to take penicillin orally for 10 days for streptococcal infections were still taking it by day 9—though the full 10-day treatment is necessary to kill all the bacteria and thus eliminate the risk of a new flare-up of infection. Only 19 per cent of a group instructed to take penicillin for recurrent rheumatic fever complied over the designated period of time.

It would seem clear that while many people may pay dearly for their medical advice, they often throw it away. One group of researchers who studied the subject developed a rule of thumb: When drugs are prescribed for the most common ills, one third of patients always take their medicines, one third sometimes take them and one third never do.

Doubts about taking a medicine will be largely eliminated if you participate actively in your interview with the doctor. But there are pitfalls in the task of following a prescription to the letter. Common ones are missing a daily dose, taking medicines at the wrong time or doubling up on an afternoon dose to make up for a missed morning one.

The hazards of this kind of error vary. A child taking antibiotics to prevent a recurrence of rheumatic fever, for example, can take as little as 30 per cent of the average prescribed dose and still be safe. An adult with high blood pressure, on the other hand, must take at least 80 per cent of the medicine, for the treatment to be effective. One missed dose of insulin could dangerously raise a diabetic's blood-sugar level, and several missed doses could lead to a coma; one missed dose of a contraceptive could lead to a pregnancy.

There are strategies you can follow to help you comply more easily with instructions. If you have to take more than one drug daily, for example, a simple calendar-like chart hung on a wall may help. With each day marked off in hours,

make a note for each pill at its appropriate time; as you take the pills, cross them off on the chart.

For a pill taken twice daily, turn the container upside down after the morning dose as a reminder to take it in the evening; then turn it right side up after taking the second dose. Or count out the pills you have to take each day and put them in a small container you can easily carry with you at home or work; but ask your pharmacist whether any of the pills will react adversely with each other or with the container.

To promote compliance, drugs for which a daily dose is absolutely essential, such as birth-control pills, are sold in special packets having the pills in separate slots either numbered consecutively or marked with the days of the week. Also available are dispensing aids *(pages 64-65)* that show the time and day of the dose last taken and of the next.

Of course, a time may come when the drug seems not to be working. If your condition has not improved by the time your doctor told you it would, call for further advice. But keep taking the drug unless and until you are told to stop.

Sometimes, however, there may be a good reason to stop taking a drug immediately—when you experience a reaction to it that threatens your health far more than the illness you have. Your doctor should warn you what changes could signal an adverse reaction. Acid indigestion and stomach distress in a patient taking phenylbutazone for bursitis, for example, could signal imminent danger of a bleeding ulcer. If any symptoms you have been warned of or other severe and unexpected side effects appear, you should ordinarily stop taking the drug and call your doctor. Even here there are exceptions, however: A patient with coronary heart disease, for example, who is taking propranolol and suddenly stops taking the drug may risk a heart attack; in the event of an adverse reaction, such a patient should keep taking the drug but get help immediately.

Although such crises in prescription-drug treatment must be guarded against, drugs save many more lives than they ever put at risk. And the more rational an approach you take to your own prescription, working closely with your doctor, the more likely it is that your own treatment will make you well and keep you healthy. ✳

Drug-making: a marvel of precision and purity

Manufacturing any pharmaceutical is a demanding task, requiring extraordinary precision, cleanliness and quality control. If the drug is an injectable—one that will be administered by hypodermic or directly into the bloodstream, circumventing such protective filters as the digestive system and skin—the job is even harder; the purity of the dose becomes a matter of life or death.

Indeed, the emphasis on purity in making injectables is so great that key areas of manufacturing plants are automated or remotely controlled, minimizing the chance of contamination. For many operations that require a human touch, personnel are cocooned in sterile coveralls, hats, boots, gloves, masks and goggles *(right)*.

In work areas, air is cleaned by filters that remove 99.97 per cent of all foreign particles, including some as small as $1/85,000$ inch. And critical portions of assembly lines, such as filling and sealing machines, are bathed in laminar air flow—streams of sterilized air that sweep away any remaining contaminants. Most equipment is stainless steel, which is easily sterilized, is noncorrosive and does not react chemically with drug compounds. As a final safety step, the rubber used for plugs is chosen for its ability to spring closed when a hypodermic needle is withdrawn—ensuring, to the extent possible, that patients receiving injections from the vial get a dose as pure as when it left the factory.

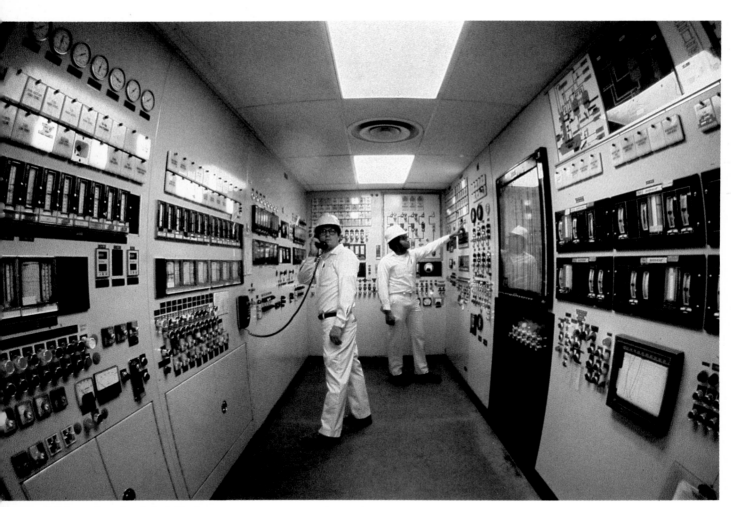

A fisheye view of an injectable-drug plant's computerized remote-control room shows rows of flashing lights, dials and recorders that provide production data for a drug being purified automatically in a distant area of the factory.

A mixing-machine operator, swathed in a sterile "bunny suit," checks a stainless-steel 1,000-gallon tank to see if it is ready for compounding an antibiotic from powdered and liquid ingredients. For sanitation, the uniform is of a lint-free synthetic.

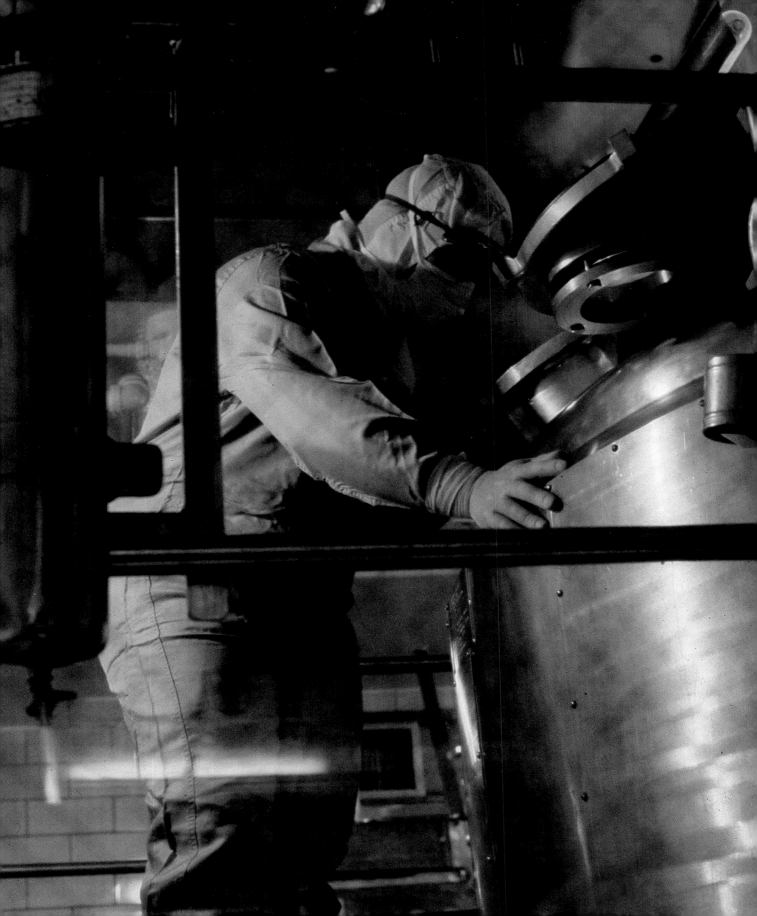

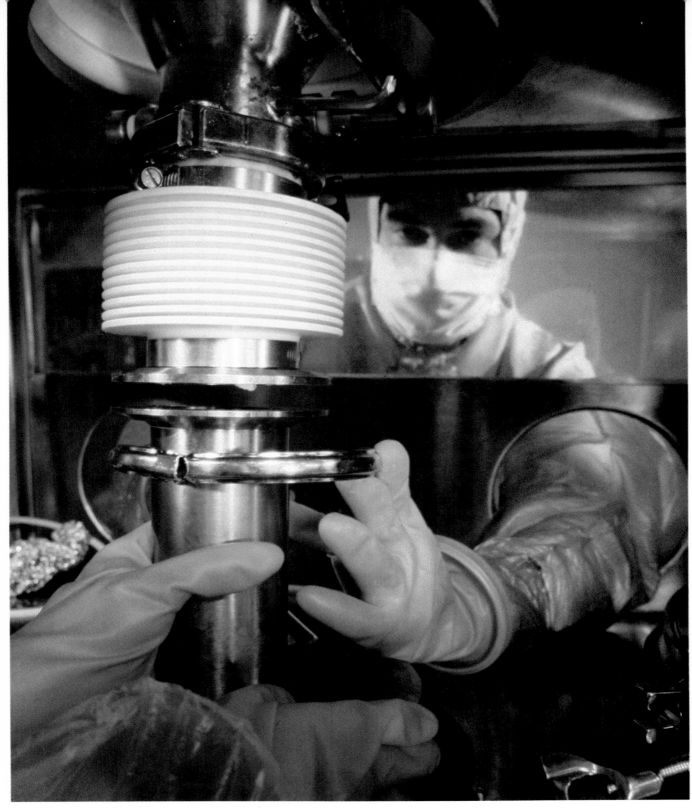

*Two technicians, working from opposite sides, reach into a
sterile chamber through built-in rubber gloves to clamp stainless-
steel pipes together. They will then transfer powdered
antibiotic from a vacuum dryer above to a container below. This
powder—the form required for injectables that deteriorate if
stored in solution—is mixed with liquid just before use.*

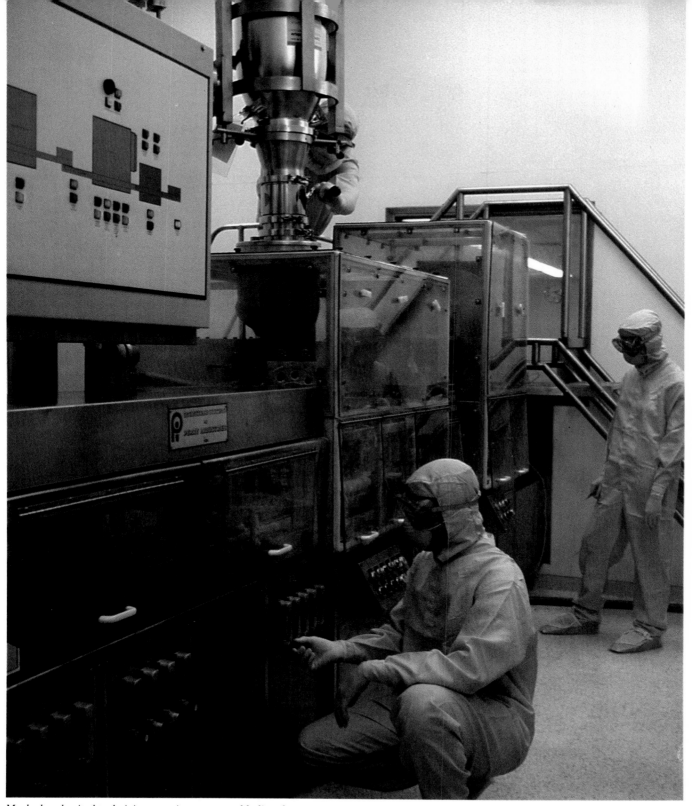

Masked and suited technicians monitor an assembly line that sterilizes, fills and plugs vials of antibiotic powder. The supervisor (foreground) adjusts a flow of nitrogen—used to flush oxygen out of the vials—while one assistant controls the flow of powder from an overhead container and another (right) stands ready to remove defective vials with sterile forceps.

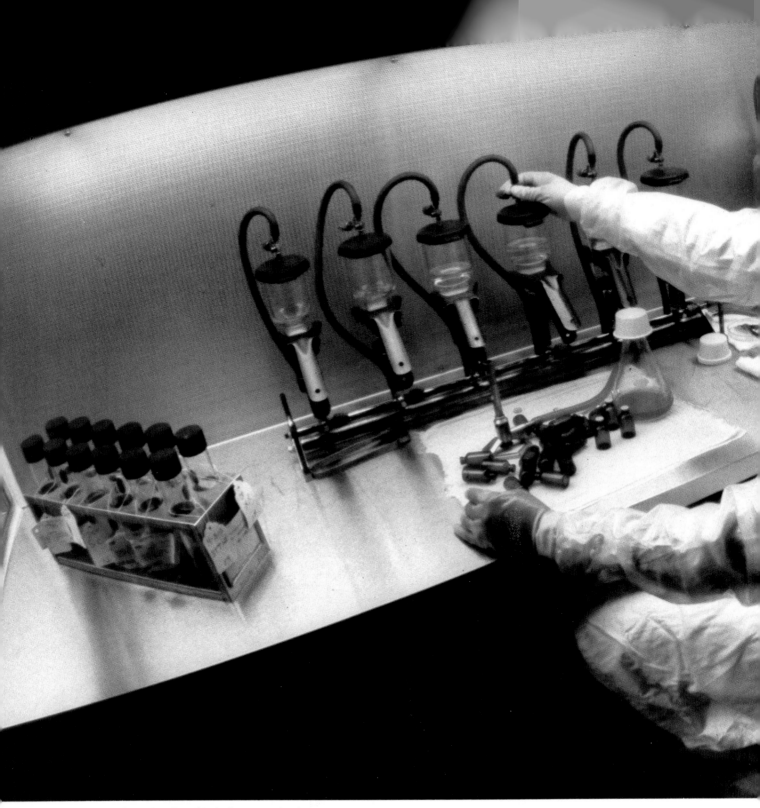

Testing vials of powdered antibiotic for contamination,
technicians force samples through filters in filtration flasks. The
filters, with pores $1/115,000$ inch in diameter, are then immersed
in tubes of culture medium (left) for up to two weeks; if the solution
turns cloudy, indicating the presence of microorganisms, the
entire batch of antibiotic is rejected.

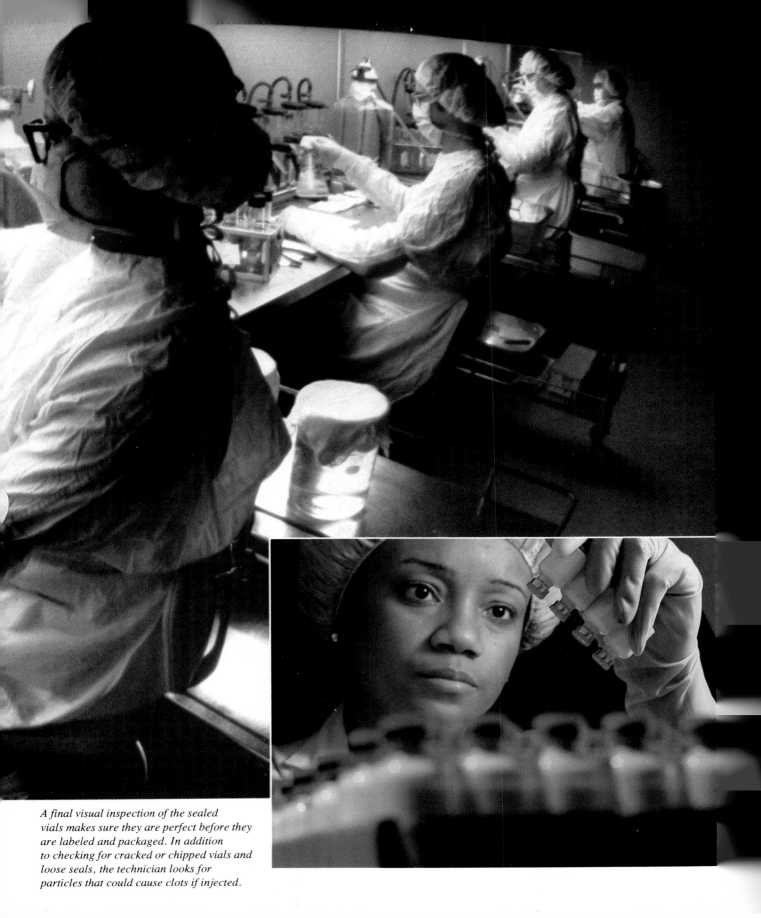

A final visual inspection of the sealed vials makes sure they are perfect before they are labeled and packaged. In addition to checking for cracked or chipped vials and loose seals, the technician looks for particles that could cause clots if injected.

CHAPTER 4

How drugs work—and sometimes don't

A frustrating search for mechanisms
Three ways chemicals cure disease
The germ-killers
Unwanted responses: the side effects
Dangerous mixtures of drugs, food and drink

The point of the cartoon on the opposite page is comic, but it has serious overtones: Knowing how medicines find their targets and do their jobs is important to everyone who uses them. Equally important—indeed, sometimes far more important—is knowing how and why they can miss their targets, with unintended and undesirable effects. Consider these case histories, in which the facts are true though the names of the participants are omitted.

● As the surgeons at a Virginia hospital started to operate on a 42-year-old woman, every sign indicated an uncomplicated procedure. Then after the first incision, the patient began to bleed profusely—and a routine operation suddenly became a life-threatening emergency. The physicians quickly gave their patient an injection of vitamin K, which promotes blood clotting, and snaked the tubing of a container of blood into a needle in her arm. Though the surgeons trying to control the bleeding did not know it, the patient had been taking large amounts of a popular painkiller for over a year; though she did not know it, the over-the-counter medicine contained aspirin, which not only kills pain but also slows blood clotting.

● An attorney had just returned from a visit to the dentist in an office near his own. A painful gum infection had been drained, and he had in his pocket a bottle of penicillin pills, prescribed by the dentist. He took the first pill. Within minutes, his hands and feet began to itch, his face swelled and he was overcome by a fit of choking and gasping. He rushed back to the dentist. There he received epinephrine and oxy-gen to counter an overwhelming allergic reaction to the antibiotic—a reaction that, untreated, could have caused a fatal collapse within minutes.

● A 61-year-old diabetic woman had a headache. She took two plain aspirin tablets along with her evening dose of tolbutamide, a medicine that controls diabetes by reducing sugar in the blood. Then she lay down to rest before dinner. When her daughter came home from work, she found her mother unconscious. A doctor, summoned at once, gave the unconscious woman an injection of glucose, which brought her back to consciousness. Her headache had been an early sign of dangerously low blood sugar. The combined action of tolbutamide and aspirin had reduced her blood sugar to a point at which she lapsed into a diabetic coma.

The very drugs that caused these terrifying effects are rightly considered modern medical wonders, but like other prescription and nonprescription medicines they can sometimes bring at least three kinds of consequences very different from those intended. For one thing, they trigger side effects, extra actions in addition to their intended ones. One of the known side effects of aspirin is a reduction in blood clotting. Side effects like this one can be predicted. The woman who nearly lost her life in a routine operation because of the anticoagulation effect of aspirin is a case in point. If she had told her doctors about her medication habits, they would have told her to stop taking the drug and would have delayed the surgery until her blood could clot normally.

A second type of drug reaction, typified by the lawyer's

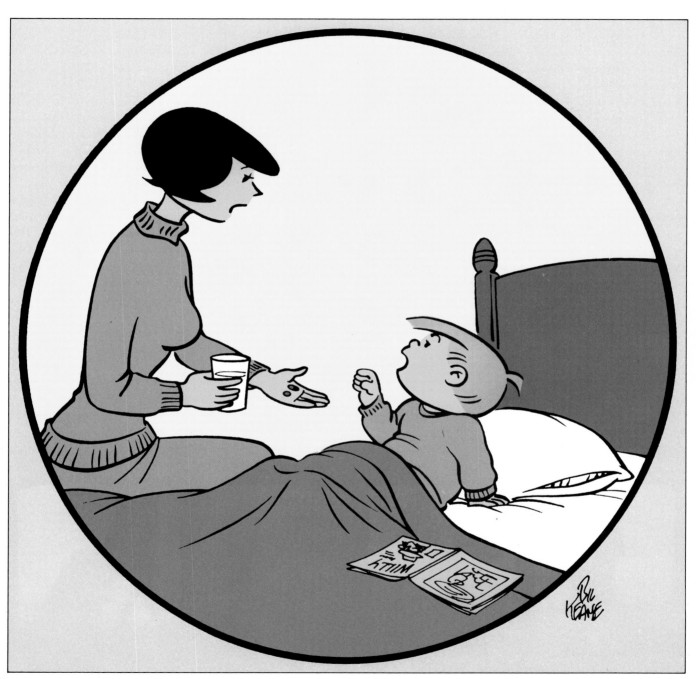

"One pill is for your sore throat; the other is for your ear ache." "How do the pills know where to go?"

near-catastrophic allergy to penicillin, is of its nature unexpected. Doctors know that some people are allergic to penicillin, but they cannot easily tell in advance who has the allergy. The adverse reaction largely depends on a victim's distinctive body chemistry, and the tools that measure body chemistry are not sufficiently sophisticated to provide an accurate prediction.

A third type of reaction arises from the interference of other substances with a drug. When several drugs are taken together, potential hazards are compounded. The human body consists of a great many chemicals, which sometimes attract one another, sometimes repel, always modifying one another's characteristics and actions. When a drug—a foreign chemical—drops into this whirlpool, the result can be profound and disturbing. The chemicals in food, beverages, alcohol and drugs may lessen or cancel the effect of a medicine. Or a drug's effects may be enhanced by another potent substance. This is what happened when the elderly diabetic took aspirin and tolbutamide together; the effect was more potent than the sum of the two drugs taken separately.

Many pharmaceutical experts who have studied drug reactions believe that negative reactions have been on the increase since the 1940s, when large numbers of new drugs began to be introduced. Certainly, research on the problem paints an ominous picture. A 1966 study of five Boston-area hospitals, headed by Dr. Dennis Slone, showed that more than 30 per cent of patients on drug treatments had adverse reactions to their medicines, and that most of these reactions were moderately severe or worse.

This grim statistic may well represent only the tip of the iceberg. The use of drugs at home multiplies the hazards, particularly when people try to treat themselves. As many as 300,000 Americans are hospitalized every year because of bad drug reactions. Part of the problem may be that drugs have become more popular today, and there are far more of them to take. Each drug type may be represented by hundreds of different products, formulated by different manufacturers in slightly different ways—and acting slightly differently.

Even the least potent drug has side effects, can cause adverse reactions in some patients and may, in combination with other substances, trigger dangerous interactions. It is difficult, and at times impossible, for a doctor to chart a perfectly safe course for every patient. At the very least, a patient can help by telling the doctor what other drugs he is taking, and by asking about possible side effects, negative reactions and interactions.

For one thing, it is necessary to make sure that the correct medicine is being taken. Doctors occasionally prescribe the wrong medicine or the wrong dose. No one knows how frequently such mistakes happen, but one small-city pharmacist whose store dispenses some 300 prescriptions every day says he sees about two wrong drugs and seven incorrect doses prescribed each week.

Even when the drug is correct and the instructions explicit,

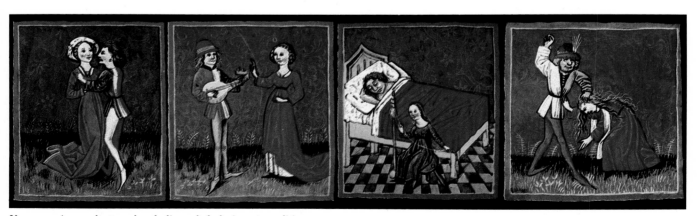

Unresponsive, ardent, melancholic and choleric personalities, portrayed (left to right) in this 15th Century German manuscript illustration, were meant to depict the four humors of ancient medicine—phlegm, blood, black bile and yellow bile. The humors were believed to be out of balance in sick people, and ancient drugs were intended to work by correcting the imbalance.

some patients forget the directions or do not understand them, or decide that since one pill is helping, taking two might work even better.

Such errors are understandably common among the elderly, many of whom must take several medicines on complex schedules. A 76-year-old man had prescriptions for five drugs from two different doctors—a sleeping pill, a drug to regulate heartbeat, a diuretic, a potassium supplement and a drug that strengthens the heart's contractions. Except for the sleeping pill, taken nightly, each medicine was meant to be administered from two to four times a day. But the patient never understood the importance of these precise schedules. All he knew for sure was that four of the medicines were for his heart, and that they were expensive. Quite independently of his doctors—neither of whom knew he was taking heart medicines prescribed by the other—he decided, as he put it, to take "one of the small pills and one of the large pills every day" in order not to use up the heart medicine too quickly. What he was doing could have led to a heart attack had it not been caught in time by a nurse.

A frustrating search for mechanisms

Old or young, any patient is better equipped to monitor his own use of medicines if he understands what drugs do in the body. This understanding has been slow in coming. Since man's first days on earth, he has experimented with the natural substances in his environment and discovered that some of them could relieve pain or other symptoms of disease. An Egyptian papyrus inscribed in 1550 B.C. recommended several medicines that are still used today—castor oil for constipation, opium as a painkiller and colchicine to treat gout.

But most early remedies did not work. They were based upon medical theories like those of the Fifth Century B.C. Greek physician Hippocrates, who believed that disease was the result of an imbalance of vital fluids: blood, phlegm, black and yellow bile. He believed that the doctor's role was merely to allow the body to heal itself. Moderation of diet, cleanliness and rest were prescribed. The drugs that were used, most of them useless, were generally mixtures of numerous ingredients, an idea later popularized by Galen, the

Greek physician of the Second Century A.D., who promulgated Hippocrates' beliefs in textbooks used for more than a thousand years. For example, a 15th Century pain mixture called Paracelsus' laudanum contained gold and pearls. Fortunately for the sufferer, the brew also contained the active painkiller opium.

Perhaps in response to the cost of concoctions like that of Paracelsus, doctors of the 16th and early 17th Centuries began experimenting with crude preparations made from a single source, such as the opium poppy. Results remained largely unpredictable and uncontrollable. As late as the 18th Century, the French satirist Voltaire summed up millennia of medical confusion in these words: "Therapeutics is the pouring of a drug of which one knows nothing into a patient of whom one knows less."

Toward the end of that century, however, the mysteries surrounding drug actions began to clear. An Italian scientist of the time, Felice Fontana, theorized that every crude drug, if effective, contained an active substance that acts on a particular area or organ of the patient. Fontana's hypothesis was borne out in 1806, when the German apothecary Friedrich Wilhelm Adam Sertürner isolated a white crystalline powder from opium. The powder was morphine, the active ingredient of crude opium *(pages 26-27),* and Sertürner's discovery created the first opportunity in human history to use a pure and active drug for medical treatment. Then in 1841, an English physician named James Blake proved that the chemical structure of a drug determines its effects on the body. At last new drugs could be tailor-made to produce specific effects in the body.

A major effort of this kind was carried out by the German bacteriologist Paul Ehrlich at the dawn of the 20th Century. In a successful search to find a compound that would cure syphilis, Ehrlich prepared and tested more than 900 compounds before he found one that worked: arsphenamine. But it was not until in the decades after World War I that the science of pharmacology reached maturity, as scientists focused in a precise way on the mechanisms responsible for a drug's effect upon particular organs and cells. Whole new classes of drugs were developed in this way. Among them were antibiotics and antihistamines, born in the 1940s. Other examples include oral contraceptives, high-blood-pressure pills and antipsychotic drugs, which arrived a decade later; and in the 1960s such drugs as antiviral medicines and L-dopa, used to treat a disorder of the nervous system called Parkinson's disease.

Getting to the target

During the long search for useful medicines, scientists found that a drug's effects depend largely on how it is absorbed, how it is distributed and transformed in the body and, finally, how it is eliminated from the body.

Absorption is the first step in the process. Before a drug can do its job, it must be broken down into molecules, which generally pass into the blood for distribution. The site and degree of absorption determine how much of a medicine acts on tissues and organs and how much of it is eliminated without change.

Normally, a drug taken by mouth takes about an hour to be absorbed by the digestive tract and passed on to the blood, to be carried elsewhere in the body. Drugs injected directly into a vein act much faster because they start their journey in the bloodstream. Injections, such as the glucose shot given to the diabetic after she lapsed into a coma, are frequently used in emergency situations.

Drugs applied to the skin, called topical drugs, may not be absorbed by the blood at all. Antiacne creams, dandruff shampoos, and medicines for athlete's foot act directly on cells at the site of application. There are exceptions to this rule. Topical nitroglycerin, used to treat the pain of heart disease, does pass into the bloodstream, and is carried by the blood to muscles of the heart.

How well and how fast an oral drug is absorbed depends on a number of factors. One of the most important is the ease with which the medicine dissolves in the acids of the stomach or the alkaline environment of the small intestine. A drug's concentration can also affect how readily it is absorbed. So can the inert materials mixed with active ingredients to form a tablet or the coating of a capsule. Thus, two manufacturers' formulations of the same medicine may be absorbed at very different rates. The drugs may be chemically equivalent—that is, made of the same amounts of an identical active ingredient—but unequal in bioavailability, because they are not available to the body at the same rate.

Once a pill dissolves in the stomach or intestines, its molecules pass into the tiny blood vessels that surround these organs. To do so, the molecules must pass through the membranes, or sheaths, of cells making up the lining of the stomach or intestines and the walls of the blood vessels. The passage can occur in three ways. Cell membranes consist partly of fat and protein molecules organized in a kind of mosaic pattern, partly of special channels for water. Small drug molecules that dissolve in water pass through the channels as water flows into the cell. Larger drug molecules, insoluble in water but soluble in fats, enter the fat of the cell membrane and come out on the other side. And drugs that do not slip through the barrier in either of these ways are helped across the membrane by special carrier substances. The drug methotrexate, for example, will bind with a specific carrier on the membrane, and the drug and carrier will move across the membrane and into the blood, where the drug is then released. The same three methods enable drug molecules to cross cell membranes not only in the stomach and intestines, but elsewhere in the body.

In most cases only a tiny percentage of a drug ever reaches its target. Some of the dose may be transformed rapidly into an inactive form; some may be excreted directly, without any chemical change, or may be distributed to tissues of the body where it is not wanted. Part of a dose may be stored in body fat, a common reservoir for foreign and potentially dangerous substances.

Finally, some drug molecules can be rendered inactive by becoming attached, or bound, to proteins circulating in the blood. The molecules of such a drug-protein combination float in the blood, too large to pass through the capillaries. Drug molecules and blood proteins bind to each other because their physical structures are complementary. Some drugs fit the proteins more precisely than others; in the language of biochemistry, they are said to have a high affinity for blood proteins. The anticoagulant dicumarol is such a drug. At least 90 per cent of each dose binds with blood proteins, becoming temporarily inactivated. After a time, some of the drug is released because the molecules of other drugs, with higher affinities for the proteins, float into the bloodstream and bump dicumarol from its protein compounds.

Three ways chemicals cure disease

How medicine floating through the blood acts upon the body was a matter of speculation for centuries. When ancient physicians brewed medicinal potions, neither they nor their patients had any clear idea why some of the medicines worked. They simply observed, for example, that fever was reduced by willow and cinchona bark, which are now known to contain ingredients that act like modern aspirin and quinine pills. The key to the mechanisms of such crude drugs could be unearthed only by a scientific understanding of disease and of normal body processes.

Quinine is effective against the fever of malaria. Physicians of an earlier day knew this fact but could not explain it. Then, in 1880, the Plasmodium parasite was identified as the cause of malaria; soon afterward, researchers proved that quinine effectively treats malarial fever because it kills the malaria "bug." It was not until 1971, however, nearly a century after aspirin came into wide use, that scientists finally discovered how it works: It inhibits the release of substances called prostaglandins, which trigger local inflammation, fever and dull throbbing pain.

As more is learned about the actions of drugs, scientists have begun to group the thousands of drug effects into a few simple categories. Different experts devise different cataloguing schemes, and no scheme fully covers all the actions of the quarter million products on the market. But the actions of the drugs most people use can be classified into three major categories. Some drugs produce their effects by acting on or in the cells of the body, as do aspirin, the tranquilizer diazepam, the painkiller morphine and thousands of other drugs. Others destroy disease organisms in the body, as quinine strikes at the Plasmodium parasite or penicillin kills staphylococcus bacteria. Finally, some drugs do not work on the large, complex molecules that make up cells and organisms, but instead combine with the relatively simple molecules of chemicals floating outside the cells of the body. Antacids act in this way when they combine in the stomach with hydrochloric acid, the villain in indigestion.

By far the most important of these categories is the first. Most drugs act on tissues rather than on invading organisms or body chemicals. Many drugs in this category work by linking with chemical structures called receptors, which are located on or in the cells and which are uniquely suited to capture a substance—in this case, a drug—with a particular chemical and physical make-up.

The concept of receptors was first worked out by the turn-of-the-century German scientist Paul Ehrlich. Ehrlich reasoned that because minute amounts of drugs often cause important physical changes, the body must use drugs very selectively, and each drug must trigger some particular action. But a minute change in the chemistry of a drug, such as the rearrangement of a few of its atoms, often changes the drug's properties. Ehrlich suggested that this happens because a drug becomes active only when attached to a receptor that it fits perfectly, as a key fits a lock. It was a revolutionary idea, one that continues to guide drug research.

A contemporary of Ehrlich's, the English physiologist J. N. Langley, took the work a step further in research on the South American arrow-poison curare, which paralyzes its victims. He showed that nicotine, the drug in tobacco, works on the same muscle-cell receptors as curare, but in a different way. Normally, nicotine causes muscle contractions. But when curare is administered along with nicotine, the nicotine action is blocked and the muscle is paralyzed.

Today it is known that two or more drugs may attach to the same receptors, with different effects. Some, like nicotine, fit the chemical lock of the receptor and turn it, stimulating an action of the cell. Others, like curare, fit the receptor and occupy it, but do not turn on the cell's activity; these drugs block receptors so that other substances cannot attach to them. The first type, called an agonist, stimulates the cell to act in a certain way; the second, called an antagonist, prevents the cell from reacting to an agonist. Either

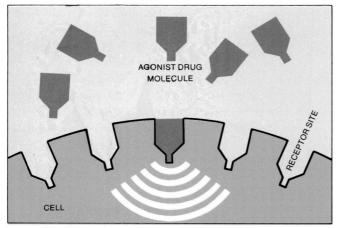

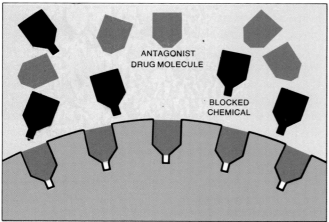

Many of the most common medicines—including some used for heart disease, allergies, ulcers and glaucoma—work because the drug compound has physical and chemical properties that "fit" a receptor site on a body cell, as diagramed above. If the drug molecule exactly fits, as the reddish molecule at top does the receptor on the cell (greenish), it is an agonist, stimulating a specific response (arcs) from the cell. If, as at bottom, the drug almost—but not quite—fits, it is an antagonist, blocking body chemicals or other drugs (black) that otherwise could produce an undesired effect on the cell.

type can make a useful remedy, one stimulating the body to throw off a disease, the other protecting the body from harmful reactions.

The germ-killers

Of the many drugs that do not act on human cells, some of the most important are aimed at foreign organisms—bacteria, viruses and parasites—that invade the body.

The great French bacteriologist Louis Pasteur was one of the first to propose that invading germs could cause disease. The idea ran counter to the prevailing dogma of his day, spontaneous generation, which held that bacteria arose from the tissue in which they were found and were not foreign to it. Pasteur, a born showman, first proved spontaneous generation false by meticulous experiments, then in 1864 drove his point home in a famous lecture given at the Sorbonne before crowds of scientists, celebrities and commoners. By sealing a sterile solution of meat extract from the germs contained in air, Pasteur had prevented new microscopic life from developing in this nutritious medium. "I wait, I watch, I question it," he cried, "begging it to recommence for me the beautiful spectacle of the first creation. But it is dumb, because I have kept it from germs which float in air, from Life, for Life is a germ and a germ is Life. Never will the doctrine of spontaneous generation recover from the mortal blow of this simple experiment."

The germ theory of disease proved productive—up to a point. Scientists developed a number of preventive vaccines and inoculations that could ward off disease. But they found no drugs to treat an infection that had taken hold upon the body—until British bacteriologist Alexander Fleming discovered penicillin, almost by accident, in 1928.

As Fleming had observed at the beginning, penicillin is virtually nontoxic. It acts solely on the bacterial cell wall, a structure that has no counterpart in animal cells. It blocks the action of a chemical that normally triggers the making of a new wall, so that the bacterial cell bursts and dies. A newer and somewhat similar antibiotic, moxalactam *(page 82),* prevents the wall from dividing in reproduction, with equally lethal results.

Not all anti-infectives work on bacterial cell walls. For example, sulfonamide drugs, used against eye and urinary-tract infections, mislead bacteria into a faulty chemical reaction that slows or stops their growth. The key to the deception is a B vitamin, folic acid, one of the building blocks of all animal and plant cells. Animals get folic acid from food, but bacteria must make their own, using an essential substance called para-aminobenzoic acid, or PABA, in a complex chemical synthesis. The sulfonamide drugs upset this synthesis. Chemically and physically similar to PABA, they take its place in the process that normally produces folic acid. Without folic acid, bacterial growth slows down; eventually it stops, and the body's immune system delivers the final blow to the stunted bacteria that remain.

In the third major type of action, drugs work not on cells or living invaders, but on chemicals—which may themselves be either products or invaders of the body. Thus, an ordinary antacid such as sodium bicarbonate neutralizes excess acid produced in the stomach; the neutralization process yields water, salt and carbon dioxide, all of which are easily eliminated from the body.

Less widely known drugs, used to cure lead, mercury and arsenic poisoning, are called chelating agents, from the Greek word *chele,* or ''claw.'' The colorful term is chemically exact: These drugs seize upon the invading molecules of a toxic metal to form a new, harmless substance. In the treatment of lead poisoning, for example, a drug called EDTA envelops the molecules of poisonous lead to form a nonpoisonous combination that, like the products of acid neutralization, can be safely excreted.

Still other drugs operate in subtler, more complex ways on chemicals that play a part in the normal processes of the body. Heparin, for example, used to prevent blood from clotting, combines with proteins involved in coagulation, forming new substances that do not participate in the process. While not entirely halted, clotting is somewhat inhibited.

Like the EDTA that is excreted along with the lead it chelates, all drugs must eventually leave the body. Indeed, considering the number of drugs many people take in a lifetime, their bodies would be a huge junkyard of drug wastes were it not for the next step in a pill's odyssey through the body. This leg of the journey, called biotransformation, changes a drug into a form that can be excreted.

For some drugs, biotransformation begins in the intestines, where substances called enzymes also control the utilization of food by starting or accelerating the processes that break it down into usable fuel. The main scene of drug transformation, however, is the liver, which contains a group of enzymes that work specifically on drugs. The amount of these enzymes may vary from person to person and partly determines the time that a drug remains active in the body of a specific individual. Liver enzymes also play a role in an individual's sensitivity to a drug. Newborn babies and young children, for example, develop these enzymes slowly, which may be the reason they are particularly susceptible to dangerous drug reactions.

Most medicines biotransformed by the liver find their way to the kidneys, where wastes are eliminated in the urine. The kidneys act as a filter, passing some drugs directly into the urine but holding others back because they have not yet been changed into a form soluble in water. Some drugs may be reabsorbed from the urine and passed back through the kidneys to the circulating blood, remaining active in the body while undergoing additional biotransformation.

Most drugs are steadily broken down and eliminated, so that additional doses must be taken every few hours. Variations in the speed at which medicines move through the body account for the fact that some drugs must be taken more frequently than others. The speed is more or less constant, however, for each drug; taking a double dose of a potent drug not only is dangerous in itself, but generally does not make up for a missed dose, nor does it put off the time when the next one should be administered.

Unwanted responses: the side effects

Life would be simpler for doctors and patients if all drugs passed neatly through a cycle of efficient absorption, health-giving action and straightforward elimination. They do not. Drugs can either miss their target or produce an undesirable response. The most familiar and best understood of these

Pseudomonas bacteria, which cause dangerous infections in burns and open wounds and are resistant to many antibiotics, multiply on a porous filter in a dish of nutrients. Moxalactam antibiotic has not yet been administered, and the bacteria are in various stages of reproduction; some, like those at bottom left, are almost ready to split in two.

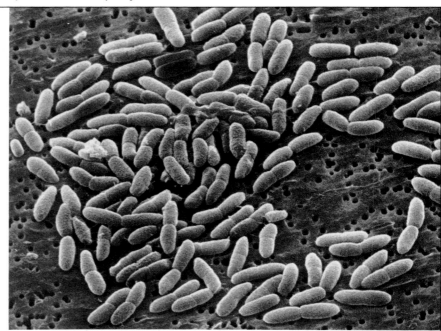

How one antibiotic makes germs commit suicide

Antibiotics have been called miracle drugs, but their ability to cure infections is no miracle. They are chemicals derived from microorganisms, and their power to kill other microorganisms is the natural outcome of biochemical reactions.

When attacking bacteria, for example, the antibiotic moxalactam—its effects are shown in the sequence of electron-microscope photographs starting at right—interferes with the growth of the bacteria's cell walls. The walls develop, but moxalactam prevents bacteria from following their normal reproduction process, in which they split in two; apparently the antibiotic suppresses a protein that normally causes the cell walls to pinch inward at the middle of a cell and form two new cells.

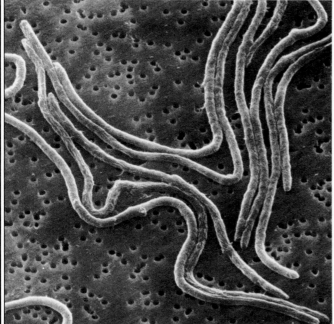

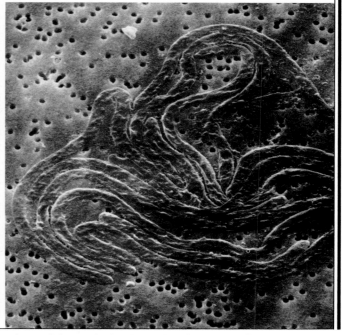

Three hours after exposure to moxalactam, the bacteria have continued to grow but they cannot divide; they are grotesquely elongated, and their weakened walls are deteriorating. In the wrinkled areas, the walls have ruptured and the innards are leaking out; the bulges are points where rupture is imminent.

After six hours, only the ghosts of the bacteria walls remain. Virtually all the contents of the bacteria have spilled out, plugging some of the filter pores. This stage represents the end of the laboratory experiment; in a human body, agents of the immune system would dissolve or carry off the bacterial debris.

unwanted responses are the side effects, which occur when the drug acts as expected but also acts on a tissue or organ other than the intended one. Typical are side effects that might affect a patient who is given a prescription drug containing pseudoephedrine to relieve the congestion and discomfort of a lingering cold. The drug will help to clear up the cold symptoms, but the patient may feel jittery and nervous for hours after taking a pill, and may not sleep well.

Pseudoephedrine constricts small blood vessels in the breathing passages of the nose and throat. As the amount of blood in these organs decreases, their tissues shrink and enlarge the passageways, making it easier for the patient to breathe. But pseudoephedrine also constricts many other blood vessels, increasing blood pressure; it stimulates the heart, increasing the rate of the pulse; and it stimulates the central nervous system. Taken together, these actions can produce the recognized side effects of pseudoephedrine: nervousness and occasional insomnia.

Because side effects are so predictable, some drugs originally designed to treat one disease are later given for another, for which the side effects are appropriate. For example, the primary—and originally the only intended—effect of diphenhydramine, an antihistamine, is the relief of allergy symptoms. Like most antihistamines, it has a side effect: drowsiness. It is sometimes prescribed for people with insomnia—and for an insomniac, the antiallergic action of the drug is the side effect.

Side effects are generally manageable. Many are transient; the nervousness of a patient who takes pseudoephedrine, for example, is generally less pronounced after a few days. And if side effects are a problem, a doctor can adjust the dose or switch to another drug. Some minor and unpleasant effects may accompany the relief conferred by any drug. The benefits may not be worth the discomforts, particularly in bearable disorders that run a definite course and go away within a limited time whether they are treated or not. The common cold, for example, usually clears up on its own in seven to 10 days. Drugs may make those days more pleasant, but they do not speed the healing process, and some people may find the side effects more unpleasant than the cold symptoms.

Since doctors know the side effects of the drugs they prescribe, they can warn patients of what to expect. In contrast, the drug effects called adverse reactions are relatively unpredictable. Fortunately, they are also relatively infrequent. But virtually anyone may have such a reaction, even under the best of circumstances—that is, even when the right drug was prescribed in the correct dose and taken under the proper conditions. What is more, the response can occur at any time. Some victims have suddenly developed drug allergies, for example, after as many as 50 years of continuous use of a particular medicine.

The reactions range from mild skin rashes, indigestion, headaches or constipation to psychotic symptoms, serious blood disorders, coma and death. They can occur instantly, in an allergic shock reaction, or over a long period of time, as in the slow deterioration of the kidneys. The effects may be brief or prolonged, reversible or permanent. Adverse reactions can even occur after a drug treatment has ended. The majority of them involve a small number of very potent drugs with a narrow safety margin—that is, with a small difference between an effective dose and a dangerous one. Such drugs are generally prescribed for illnesses that are themselves life-threatening, so that the risk of a reaction is balanced by the more serious risks of the disease.

An allergic reaction to penicillin is perhaps the best known of these events, but many drugs can provoke allergic reactions and even good doctors cannot always predict their occurrence or course. White House press secretary James Brady, for example, who sustained severe head wounds during an assassination attempt on President Ronald Reagan, developed a high allergy fever in response to dosages of anticonvulsion and blood-pressure medicines; his fever went down promptly when the drugs were changed.

In another kind of adverse reaction, called an extension reaction, allergy is not involved. The organs and cells of the body react to the drug exactly as they are supposed to, but to an excessive degree. For example, a dose of insulin that is designed to lower a diabetic's blood sugar to a safe level may produce dangerously low blood sugar or even unconsciousness. By contrast, a so-called paradoxical reaction produces

Drugs and athletics—a losing combination

"I'm not about to go out there one-on-one against a guy who is grunting and drooling and coming at me with big, dilated pupils unless I'm in the same condition," said one professional football player, defending his drug use in the late 1960s. His team, the San Diego Chargers *(below),* then took some 10,000 stimulants, sedatives, painkillers and other drugs yearly to improve performance.

Drug abuse among athletes is not limited to football—or to professional sports. One American track coach has estimated that 70 per cent of all United States amateur track-and-field stars have used anabolic steroids, the male sex-hormone derivatives.

But many drug takers find their performance is not improved and may be impaired; others aggravate old injuries or suffer new

ones. Houston Ridge, a former defensive lineman with the Chargers, claimed that the drugs distributed in the locker room made him more vulnerable to the hip injury that ended his career in 1969. Baseball player Jim Palmer *(right, bottom)* got a skin burn from using the anti-inflammatory drug DMSO on his pitching arm. And East Germany's Renate Vogel-Heinrich *(right, top),* a world-champion swimmer, developed Amazonian shoulders and a husky voice from a 10-year regimen of anabolic steroids.

Many experts now think the short-term benefits of sports drugs do not justify the long-term hazards. "A normal, well-fed human being," said Dr. Donald Cooper, once an Olympic-team doctor, "can never be safely improved upon by any drug."

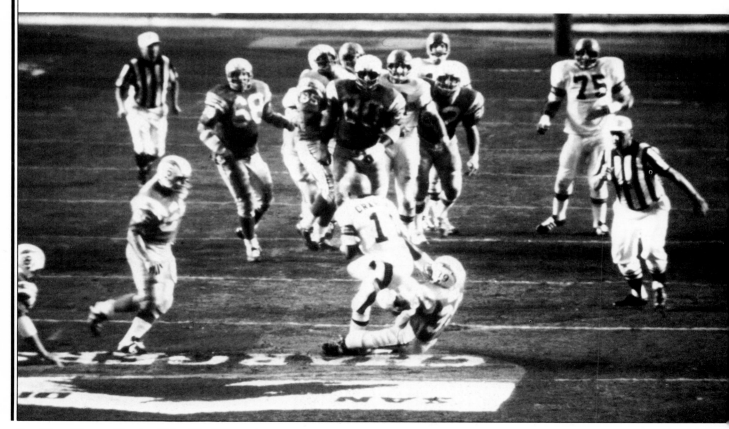

San Diego Charger Houston Ridge (No. 80) watches a teammate make a tackle in a 1969 game. Ridge won $260,000 in the 1973 settlement of a malpractice suit, arguing successfully that a career-ending hip injury was both caused and aggravated by drugs that were given to him by team officials.

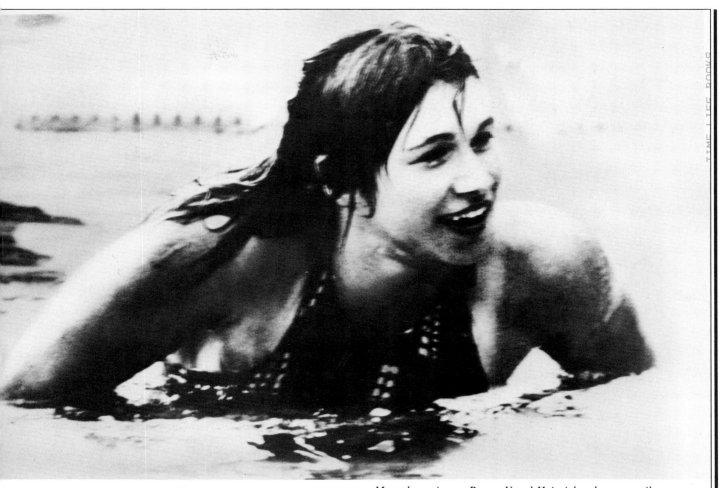

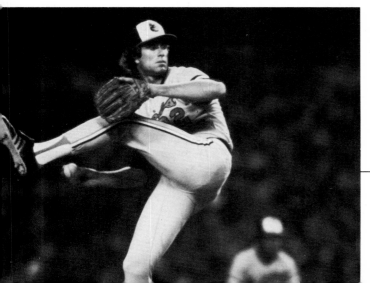

Muscular swimmer Renate Vogel-Heinrich, who won a silver medal for East Germany at the 1972 Olympics, savors a record-breaking breast-stroke performance two years later. She attributed her success to her country's system of turning out winners as "production out of a nationalized factory." But Vogel-Heinrich defected in 1979 after discovering that the factory was powered, in part, by long-term doses of steroids.

Baltimore Orioles pitcher Jim Palmer kicks and throws toward home plate. Palmer sustained an unsightly skin burn—"people asked if I had ringworm," he grumbled—from the drug DMSO. Other side effects were foul breath and body odor.

the exact opposite of a drug's expected results. Some patients who are given small doses of diazepam tranquilizer to soothe and relax them become angry and hostile, in a response that persists until the drug is stopped.

Some adverse reactions arise from genetic differences. About 10 per cent of American blacks, for example, lack an enzyme that is normally present in red blood cells. This deficiency causes their red cells to disintegrate when exposed to a wide variety of drugs, resulting in anemia. Among the drugs that are dangerous to these blacks are the anti-infective sulfonamide drugs, the gout medicine probenecid and nitrofurantoin, an antibacterial drug that normally cures some urinary-tract infections.

A final category of reactions may not be directly dangerous to the patient but can affect his treatment. Because drugs change the internal chemistry of the body, they can affect the findings of diagnostic tests designed to measure this chemistry. A false test can fail to reveal a real illness; conversely, it can make a healthy person appear sick, leading to treatment for a nonexistent malady.

Drugs may either distort a test measurement or change the level of the substance being measured. Methenamine mandelate, a drug used to treat kidney and bladder infections, can falsify urine tests for a certain hormone by indicating higher levels of the hormone than actually exist. Diuretics, which increase urine volume and are prescribed for high blood pressure, can alter the concentration of electrolytes—inorganic ions in blood and urine that aid in maintaining the metabolic process. This electrolyte imbalance may wrongly suggest that a patient has a kidney malfunction.

Dangerous mixtures of drugs, food and drink

Some of the greatest drug hazards come not from the action of an individual drug, but from a mixture of potent chemicals in the body. Medicines are the most obvious of the interacting substances, but they are not the only ones; alcohol and certain foods can combine with drugs to affect body chemistry in a harmful way.

Because there are so many possible combinations of drugs, food and drink, potential interactions often are overlooked. When an elderly patient was admitted to a hospital with a case of acute bronchitis, he was given tetracycline, an antibiotic, to cure the bacterial infection of his lungs. But because hospital tests also showed that he was slightly anemic and had an ulcer, he was given antacids to neutralize the stomach acid that activated the ulcer, and iron pills to help build up red blood cells against the anemia.

A week later it appeared that the ulcer was healing. But the patient's bronchitis was no better and he was still anemic. The antibiotic was combining with chemicals in the antacid and iron pills to form substances that could not be absorbed. Neither the tetracycline nor the iron pills were acting in adequate amounts to do their jobs.

This patient's experience was doubly unfortunate because, like many drug interactions, it resulted from known and predictable chemical reactions and could have been avoided. The doctors need only have given the drugs at different times of the day.

But not all interactions can be prevented so easily. Like adverse reactions to single drugs, some interactions are linked to a patient's individual body chemistry as determined by such factors as age, sex, heredity, and by changes brought about by illness or the long use of medicines. Some harmful interactions well known to doctors occur in only a few patients—an example is that between the sedative phenobarbital and the anticonvulsion medicine diphenylhydantoin, which may aggravate the pattern of epileptic seizures in some patients. In most cases, mixing these drugs causes no harm. Indeed the sedative may contribute to the control of epileptic seizures. In such instances, a doctor may choose to risk the potentially dangerous combination of drugs if an interaction is rare, if the drugs are necessary and, above all, if no medication alternatives are available.

Medicines can combine to produce a variety of effects. In one type of interaction, one drug may enhance the effects of another, sometimes to a great extent. Such an interaction, called synergism, can be very dangerous. Some unwary patients, for example, have taken aspirin along with warfarin, an anticoagulant. Aspirin, too, delays blood clotting, and the combined effect of both drugs—far greater than the sum of the individual effects—may be uncontrollable bleeding.

In an opposite interaction, drugs lessen or even eliminate each other's effects. When a barbiturate sleeping pill or sedative is taken with an antihistamine, the antiallergic action of the antihistamine may be reduced; the barbiturate can speed its elimination from the body by enhancing the action of drug-metabolizing enzymes in the liver. Tetracycline and penicillin, both antibiotics, are an equally poor combination; tetracycline inhibits penicillin's action against the growth of bacterial cell walls.

A single substance can, in different mixtures, have both synergistic and suppressive effects. The worst offender is alcohol, which plays a part in some of the most common—and most dangerous—of all interactions. Of the hundred most frequently prescribed drugs, about half contain at least one ingredient that reacts badly with alcohol. Every year, some 47,000 people who have taken drugs when drinking are treated in hospital emergency rooms, and more than 2,500 die from the combination.

Alcohol depresses central nervous system activity and, when mixed with drugs that do the same thing, may produce a profoundly synergistic effect. Drowsiness can increase, judgment and alertness can be impaired, the victim may have trouble walking, talking, driving and thinking. The result may even be death; when a barbiturate is taken along with alcohol, the amount that ordinarily would be required to kill a person is reduced by half.

On the other hand, the chronic use of excessive alcohol can diminish the effects of other drugs. Alcoholics sometimes need 50 per cent more than the normal dosages of such drugs as tolbutamide, a diabetes remedy; phenytoin, an anticonvulsion drug; warfarin, the anticoagulant; and isoniazid, used to treat tuberculosis.

Interactions between drugs and food are numerous, but their effects are usually mild. Occasionally, however, such combinations can cause serious harm. Diets rich in dairy products may diminish the effect of digitalis, a heart medication, by interfering with the drug's absorption. Large amounts of licorice can raise blood pressure to such a degree that high-blood-pressure remedies no longer work. Antico-

A personal medical warning system

Medical identification such as an inscribed bracelet *(below)* or wallet card can save the life of anyone afflicted by a chronic ailment that is not obvious—such as heart disease, allergies, diabetes or epilepsy. If he should be unable to communicate in an emergency, the identification provides information for appropriate first aid and protection against possibly harmful treatment.

Several organizations offer medical identification services. One of the most popular is provided by the Medic Alert Foundation International of Turlock, California, an association with nearly two million members in more than a dozen countries. Each member gets a bracelet or necklace engraved with the owner's health problem, an identification number and the telephone number of Medic Alert's emergency answering service. At a glance, a rescuer recognizing the tag of an unconscious person has a head start in diagnosis and treatment and, by dialing the number, can obtain a medical history from the file that Medic Alert keeps on every member.

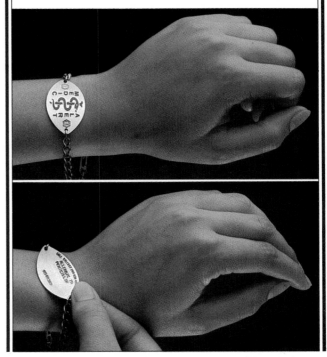

The face of a Medic Alert identification tag (top) bears the internationally recognized staff and snake insignia of the medical profession. The other side of the tag describes the wearer's medical problem—in this case, a penicillin allergy. It also gives a phone number and a membership number, so that rescue or hospital personnel can obtain further medical information.

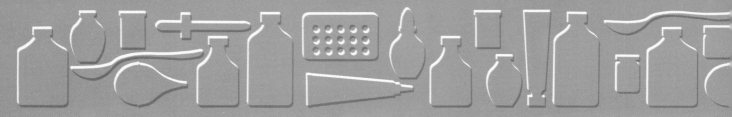

Avoiding dangerous drug interactions

Almost any medicine can interact with any other to cause ill effects—tranquilizers, other nerve depressants and the heart medicine warfarin are among the notorious offenders. Consult your doctor before taking these drugs with any others. Some other medicines, commonly used but less widely recognized for their hazards of interaction, are listed below.

The 44 prescription (Rx) and nonprescription drugs in the list are identified by the generic chemical names of their active ingredients, with common brand names underneath. To use the table, identify the active ingredient of the medicine—check the label or ask the pharmacist—then note and avoid the drugs and foods with which it interacts.

ALUMINUM HYDROXIDE
Amphojel, Delcid, Di-Gel, Gelusil
Interferes with the antibiotic tetracycline, the tranquilizer chlorpromazine and isoniazid, used for tuberculosis; take them at least 3 hours apart.

AMINOPHYLLINE (Rx)
Aminodur, Somophyllin
Effects may be reduced by the high-blood-pressure drug propranolol. Effects may be intensified by cimetidine, used for ulcers.

AMITRIPTYLINE (Rx)
Elavil, Endep
Reduces effects of clonidine and guanethidine, used for high blood pressure. May produce elevated blood pressure and irregular heartbeat if taken with phenylephrine, a nasal decongestant, or epinephrine, used for heart disease, glaucoma or asthma. May reduce effects of anticonvulsant drugs used to treat epilepsy.

ASPIRIN
Many brand names
Reduces effects of probenecid and sulfinpyrazone, used for gout.

CALCIUM CARBONATE
Titralac, Tums
Interferes with actions of the antibiotic tetracycline, drugs containing iron for anemia, and chlorpromazine tranquilizer; take them at least 3 hours apart.

CHLORDIAZEPOXIDE (Rx)
Librium
Effects and side effects may be intensified by cimetidine, a drug that controls ulcers.

CHLOROTHIAZIDE (Rx)
Diuril
Intensifies side effects of lithium, a tranquilizer; potassium loss caused by chlorothiazide may increase side effects of digoxin, used for heart-rhythm disorders. Potassium loss may be intensified by corticosteroids used to reduce inflammation.

CHLORPROMAZINE (Rx)
Promapar, Thorazine
Effects may be reduced by aluminum hydroxide and other antacids. Some side effects—dry mouth, constipation and difficulty urinating—may be intensified by imipramine and other drugs used to treat depression. May reduce effects of levodopa, used for Parkinson's disease, and guanethidine, used for high blood pressure.

CHLORPROPAMIDE (Rx)
Diabinese
Effects may be inhibited by thiazides, drugs used for high blood pressure, and by epinephrine, used for heart disease or asthma. Effects may be intensified by the following: aspirin; clofibrate, a cholesterol reducer; chloramphenicol, an antibiotic; phenylbutazone, a painkiller that reduces inflammation; propranolol, used for high blood pressure and heart disease; and thyroid hormone.

CIMETIDINE (Rx)
Tagamet
May intensify effects and side effects of propranolol, used for heart disease and high blood pressure, and of the tranquilizers chlordiazepoxide, clorazepate and diazepam.

CLORAZEPATE (Rx)
Tranxene
Interactions similar to CHLORDIAZEPOXIDE

CORTISONE (Rx)
Cortone
Decreases the effects of drugs used to treat diabetes. Potassium loss caused by cortisone increases side effects of digoxin and digitoxin, drugs used for heart-rhythm disorders. May increase risk of ulcer if taken with aspirin or other drugs that reduce inflammation.

DIAZEPAM (Rx)
Valium
Effects and side effects may be intensified by cimetidine, a drug that controls ulcers.

DIGITOXIN (Rx)
Crystodigin
Side effects may be intensified by cortisone, a drug that reduces inflammation, and by quinidine, used for heart-rhythm disorders.

DIGOXIN (Rx)
Lanoxin, SK-Digoxin
Interactions similar to DIGITOXIN

DISULFIRAM (Rx)
Antabuse
May intensify the effects and side effects of phenytoin, used for epilepsy. May produce radical mental changes if taken with isoniazid, a tuberculosis drug, or with metronidazole, a drug used to treat vaginitis.

DOXYCYCLINE (Rx)
Vibramycin
Effects may be reduced by antacids, dairy products and drugs containing iron for anemia; take them at least 3 hours apart.

EPHEDRINE
Azma-Aid, Quibron
May produce dangerous rise in blood pressure if taken with phenelzine, used for depression. May decrease effects of guanethidine, used for high blood pressure.

ERYTHROMYCIN (Rx)
Erythrocin, Pediazole
May intensify effects and side effects of theophylline, a drug used to treat asthma.

ETHINYL ESTRADIOL (Rx)
Estinyl, Norlestrin
May alter effects of drugs for diabetes. May decrease

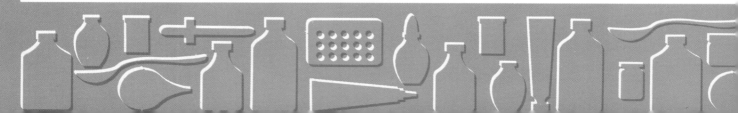

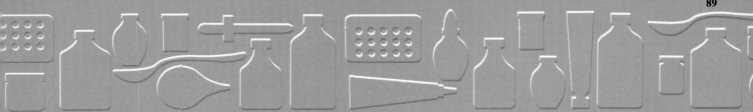

effects of clofibrate, used to lower cholesterol levels.

FENOPROFEN (Rx)
Nalfon
Increases likelihood of stomach ulcers if taken with large amounts of aspirin or other drugs used for inflammation.

FERROUS FUMARATE (Rx), FERROUS GLUCONATE (Rx), FERROUS SULFATE (Rx)
Fergon, Fero-Gradumet, Hemocyte
Effects may be inhibited by antacids and by the antibiotic tetracycline; take them at least 3 hours apart.

IBUPROFEN (Rx)
Mortin
Interactions similar to FENOPROFEN

LEVODOPA (Rx)
Bendopa, Dopar, Larodopa
Effects may be reduced by the following: vitamin B6; phenytoin, used for epilepsy; chlorpromazine, a tranquilizer; papaverine, used to treat circulatory disorders; and clonidine, used to treat high blood pressure.

LITHIUM (Rx)
Eskalith, Lithonate
Effects may be reduced by aminophylline and theophylline, used for asthma, and by sodium bicarbonate, an antacid.

MAGNESIUM HYDROXIDE
Delcid, Di-Gel, Gelusil
May interfere with actions of the antibiotic tetracycline, drugs containing iron for anemia, and chlorpromazine for psychosis; take at least 3 hours apart.

METRONIDAZOLE (Rx)
Flagyl
May produce confusion and mental changes if taken with disulfiram, used to treat alcoholism.

OXYPHENBUTAZONE (Rx)
Oxalid, Tandearil
Increases side effects of phenytoin, used for epilepsy, and of drugs used to treat diabetes. Risk of ulcers increases if drug is taken with aspirin or other drugs used for inflammation.

PENICILLIN G & V
Pentids, V-Cillin K
Effects may be reduced by antacids containing aluminum hydroxide, and by the antibiotics chloramphenicol, erythromycin and tetracycline. Effects and side effects may be increased by probenecid, used for gout.

PENTOBARBITAL (Rx)
Nembutal
Reduces effects of cortisone, used to reduce inflammation, and of the antibiotics doxycycline and quinidine, used for heart-rhythm disorders.

PHENELZINE (Rx)
Nardil
May cause a dangerous rise in blood pressure when taken with the following: narcotics; guanethidine, used for high blood pressure; levodopa, used for Parkinson's disease; foods and beverages containing tyramine, such as chicken liver, dairy products and meats prepared with tenderizers.

PHENOBARBITAL (Rx)
Luminal
Interactions similar to PENTOBARBITAL

PHENOLPHTHALEIN
Alophen, Ex-Lax, Phenolax
May cause stomach or intestinal irritation if taken with antacids or milk.

PHENYTOIN (Rx)
Dilantin
Effects and side effects may be increased by chloramphenicol, an antibiotic; disulfiram, used for alcoholism; isoniazid, a tuberculosis drug; and phenylbutazone, a painkiller. Effects may be reduced by drugs used to treat depression, such as amitriptyline.

POTASSIUM (Rx)
Kaon, Kay Ciel, Slow-K
Salt substitutes containing potassium may increase side effects of this drug. Triamterene and spironolactone, two drugs used for high blood pressure, may also increase its side effects.

PREDNISONE (Rx)
Deltasone, Orasone
Interactions similar to CORTISONE

PROCHLORPERAZINE (Rx)
Combid, Compazine
Effects may be reduced by antacids, and by benztropine and trihexyphenidyl, used for Parkinson's disease. Intensifies side effects of drugs used to treat depression. May reduce effects of levodopa, used for Parkinson's disease, and of guanethidine, used for high blood pressure.

PROPRANOLOL (Rx)
Inderal
Effects and side effects may be intensified by cimetidine, used to control ulcers. Propranolol may interfere with effects of drugs used to treat diabetes and with isoproterenol, used for asthma. If taken with aminophylline or theophylline, used for treating asthma, effects of each drug may be reduced.

QUINIDINE (Rx)
Quinaglute, Quinidex, Quinora
Effects may be reduced by phenytoin, used for epilepsy. Effects and side effects of this drug may be intensified by acetazolamide, used to treat glaucoma. Intensifies effects and side effects of digoxin, used to control heart-rhythm disorders.

SULFISOXAZOLE (Rx)
Gantrisin, Pediazole
May increase effects and side effects of phenytoin, used for epilepsy, and of drugs used to treat diabetes.

TETRACYCLINE (Rx)
Achromycin, Sumycin
Interactions similar to DOXYCYCLINE

THYROID (Rx)
Armour Thyroid
Reduces effects of drugs used to treat diabetes, such as insulin.

TRIMETHOPRIM/SULFAMETHOXAZOLE (Rx)
Bactrim, Septra
Intensifies effects and side effects of phenytoin, used for epilepsy, and of drugs used to treat diabetes.

VALPROIC ACID (Rx)
Depakene
Reduces or increases effects of phenytoin, used for epilepsy.

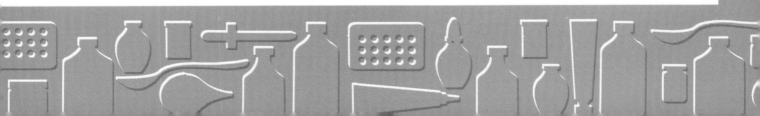

agulants can be compromised by large amounts of vitamin K, found in liver and leafy green vegetables. Other vegetables, such as soybeans, rutabagas, turnips, kale and cabbage, can counteract thyroid medicines because they block the utilization of iodine.

All these types of interactions can take place at almost any stage of a drug's passage through the body—during absorption, distribution, biotransformation or excretion. Some important interactions, especially with food, occur while a drug is being absorbed. One drug may combine with another in the digestive tract in a way that renders both ineffective. Even without a direct chemical interaction, one drug can affect the absorption of another by speeding up the digestive process or slowing it down. Laxatives, for example, tend to move drugs through the body quickly, thus shortening the period during which the drugs are in contact with the absorbing surface of the intestine; there is less time for the drug molecules to pass into the blood before they are eliminated. Other drugs, including codeine and morphine, can slow digestion and thus increase drug absorption.

Alcohol, too, can play a part here, as it does in so many interactions. It can, for example, dissolve the coating of time-released pills, accelerating their absorption and flooding the body with an excessive dose of the drug.

Even when a drug is absorbed normally, its effects may be increased or decreased by other chemicals that enhance or limit its distribution. Medicines that affect the permeability of cell membranes can change the speed at which other drugs flow through these barriers. Or a disruption of normal drug distribution can occur when a person takes two drugs, both of which act by binding with blood proteins. One diabetic patient regularly took tolbutamide to lower his blood sugar level. Because he also suffered from joint pains, his doctor decided to treat him with a painkiller, phenylbutazone. Within 24 hours his heartbeat became rapid and he began to sweat profusely. The diagnosis was simple: a dangerously low level of blood sugar. The cause was a complex interference with the distribution of tolbutamide, which is normally stored in the bloodstream. In this patient's blood, the new drug had displaced the tolbutamide from the protein storage sites that would otherwise have released it gradually and gently. In effect, the diabetic was showing the effects of a tolbutamide overdose.

In another form of molecular warfare affecting distribution in the body, drugs may compete for cell receptors. In one such case, a patient was taking guanethidine to combat high blood pressure. He was also given an antidepressant for mild depression, and within a day developed a severe headache—in his condition, the sign of an increase in blood pressure. The antidepressant had taken over crucial receptors, blocking the first drug and canceling its effect. The guanethidine never reached the cells that were its target. Though his doctor immediately stopped administering the antidepressant and raised the guanethidine dosage, it took six days for the patient's blood pressure to return to normal.

Interactions also occur during the biotransformation process that prepares drugs for elimination. Some medications combined with alcohol stimulate the liver to produce more of the enzymes responsible for the most important stages of biotransformation. When the amount of liver enzymes is increased, drugs may break down so rapidly that they do not stay in the body long enough to do much good. Hundreds of medicines, including painkillers, anesthetics, antihistamines, anti-inflammatory drugs, sedatives, tranquilizers and diabetes pills can interact with alcohol in this way. The sedative phenobarbital, for example, can accelerate the biotransformation of drugs such as digitoxin, diphenylhydantoin and griseofulvin.

Even at the final stage of drug processing, when a medicine's breakdown products are about to be eliminated, the presence of another potent substance can reverse the normal process and cause reabsorption of the drug. For example, one drug may reduce the solubility of another, so that the second drug is not taken up in the urine. Reabsorption is fairly common and not necessarily dangerous, but it does have its hazards. A combination of the painkiller phenylbutazone with the antidiabetes drug acetohexamide, taken to lower blood sugar, creates one such hazard. The painkiller can block the excretion of hydroxyhexamide, the final breakdown product of the diabetes drug. Because hydroxyhexamide retains the power to lower blood sugar, its reabsorption can cause a dangerously low sugar level.

Adverse drug reactions and interactions are complex and potentially dangerous because so many different factors bring them about. But when you must take medicines, you can find a safe course through this maze in two ways: by making the most of the knowledge and experience of your doctor and pharmacist, and by making yourself aware of the reactions that pose a real danger.

Always inform your doctor and pharmacist of all the drugs you are taking, including nonprescription remedies. Be sure you understand exactly when and how you should take a prescribed drug, and what its normal side effects are. Ask your doctor, too, whether there are foods or drugs you should avoid, and whether alcohol presents special hazards to you.

The table on pages 88-89, which lists interactions of potentially troublesome drugs, can help you recognize a dangerous reaction. Most threatening drug reactions fall into a few categories, and you can generally detect the symptoms of almost all of them. Allergic reactions to antibiotics, for example, often start with itching and swelling, while other drug allergies cause rashes or high fever. If you are diabetic, learn to recognize the effects of drug combinations that trigger dangerously low blood sugar: a rapid heartbeat, profuse sweating and a lightheaded feeling. And if you are taking a monoamine oxidase inhibitor as an antidepressant, be on the alert for a very severe headache, a possible sign of a reaction so extreme that it can cause a stroke or a heart attack.

Whenever you think you are experiencing an unexpected drug reaction, call your doctor or pharmacist immediately; if you are experiencing severe symptoms, go to the nearest hospital emergency room. Reactions that are not emergencies can be handled in discussions with your doctor or pharmacist. It may be that the dosage of the drug you are taking, or the drug itself, should be changed. Do not, however, take it upon yourself to abandon a medicine prescribed for such life-threatening conditions as diabetes, heart disease or high blood pressure, particularly if your reaction is minor: The new hazards you create may be greater than the old ones that you are trying to avoid.   ❋

Where to find the warnings

Every medicine comes with clear instructions telling how much of the drug to use, and how often, to get the intended effect. But drugs have unintended effects as well, and manufacturers are bound by law to warn users against these effects. For some prescription drugs, the warnings come in leaflets called Patient Package Inserts; for over-the-counter drugs, the place to look is in the fine print on the label or in special instructions included in the package. In all three places, the manufacturer tells the patient about the nature of a drug's side effects, the dangers of harmful interactions with other drugs and—surprisingly—the possibility that the drug may be inappropriate for the very ailment it is meant to help.

Sometimes the cautions are stated directly. The warning for a popular decongestant, for example, reads in part: "Reduce dosage if nervousness, dizziness, sleeplessness, nausea or headache occur." This is a straightforward list of side effects, along with a clear direction for one way to lessen them. The next sentence also refers to a side effect, but in an indirect way: "Individuals with high blood pressure, heart disease, diabetes, urinary retention, glaucoma or thyroid disease should use only as directed by a physician." This product works by constricting blood vessels, not only in stuffed-up nasal passages, but everywhere in the body. The side effect caused by the general constriction is a rise in blood pressure—and such a rise is potentially dangerous to sufferers from the ailments listed by the manufacturer.

Finally, there are warnings that must be read with special care to grasp their full meaning. The label on a best-selling cough syrup warns against using the product "where cough is accompanied by excessive secretions." The manufacturer is advising the patient not to try to suppress a so-called productive cough, which helps rid the body of mucus and harmful matter in the throat and lungs. Though the syrup can soothe a dry, nonproductive cough, its suppressant effect on a productive one hampers the body's effort to heal itself.

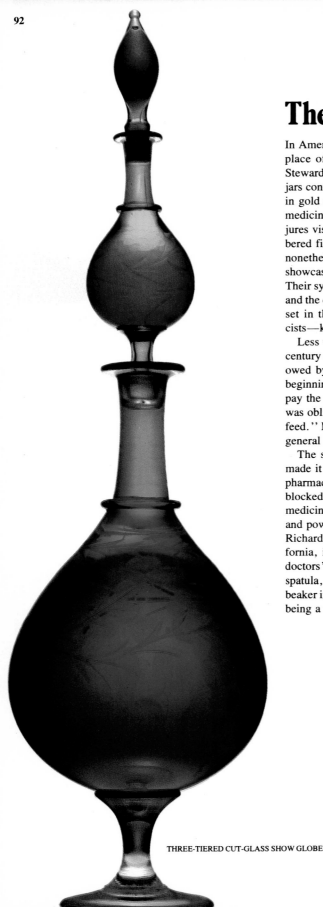

THREE-TIERED CUT-GLASS SHOW GLOBE

The drugstore of fond memory

In America at the turn of the century, the corner drugstore was a place of wonder—a neighborhood emporium, wrote historian Steward H. Holbrook, "of tremendous old wide-mouthed glass jars containing raw drugs, shelf upon shelf of them, each labeled in gold and black with the arcane Latin abbreviations of classic medicine." Nowadays the very phrase "corner drugstore" conjures visions of a bygone era. The stores themselves are remembered firsthand by a diminishing few, but are recalled distinctly nonetheless for their mahogany cabinets and glistening glass showcases, for their mirrored walls and pungent, exotic smells. Their symbols were familiar and reassuring: the mortar and pestle and the decorative show globe *(left),* filled with colored water and set in the window. Their proprietors—trusted local pharmacists—knew customers by name and medical histories by heart.

Less well recalled, however, is the fact that in the turn-of-the-century drugstore—as in the modern one—drugs were overshadowed by other commerce. The soda fountain, though it had its beginnings in medication, became a social gathering place. To pay the rent, noted Holbrook, the American pharmacist of 1900 was obliged to "deal in almost everything except hay, grain and feed." Many drugstores, in fact, more closely resembled frontier general stores than medical-supply centers.

The soul of the oldtime drugstore—indeed, the feature that made it a drugstore—was seldom seen by the public. It was the pharmacist's retreat—either a concealed back room or an area blocked from view by a high counter—where he went to make medicines. Redolent with the heady fragrance of a hundred herbs and powders, it was "a mysterious, fascinating place," recalled Richard Armour, whose father ran a pharmacy in Pomona, California, in the early 1900s. "Druggists miraculously deciphered doctors' handwriting, mixed compounds with mortar, pestle and spatula, and poured disease-curing potions from one graduated beaker into another." There, he continued, "a druggist, instead of being a merchant, was a chemist, a man of science."

The natty staff of Schroeder's Pharmacy in Quincy, Illinois, steps outside for the photographer in the 1880s. With bold-lettered signs and a mortar and pestle over the door, Schroeder's façade was typical of contemporary American drugstores. The pharmacy's other symbolic mortar and pestle, atop a curbside lamppost that doubled as a hitching post, was more unusual.

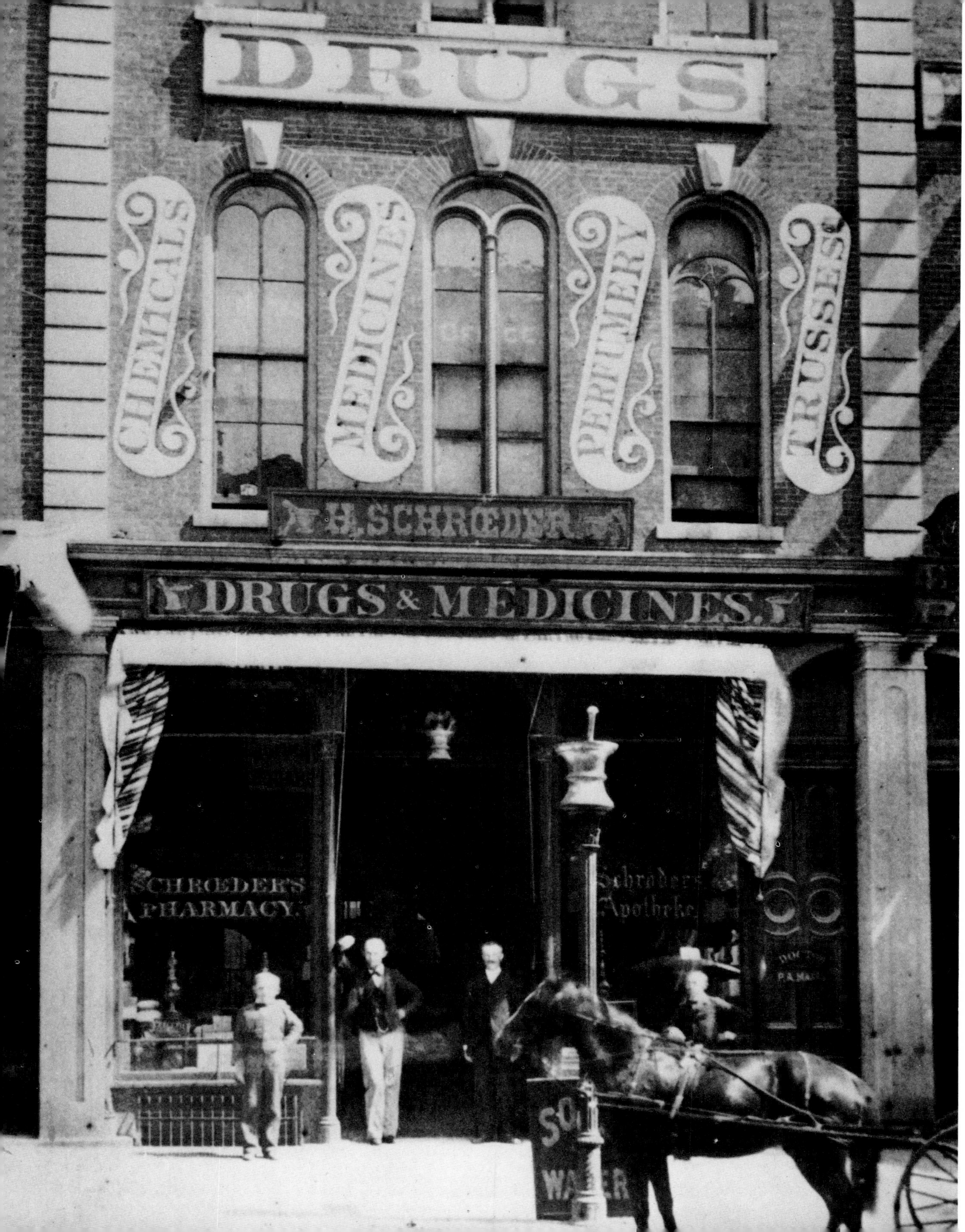
DRUGS
CHEMICALS
MEDICINES
PERFUMERY
TRUSSES
H. SCHRŒDER
DRUGS & MEDICINES
SCHRŒDER'S PHARMACY.
Schröder's Apotheke

The lure of beguiling displays

The traditional drugstore's front window was a kind of three-dimensional catalogue. There, eye-catching displays of medicines and sundries were coupled with visual reminders of the pharmacist's special skills—such as a scale used to weigh drug powders—or with decorative items meant for display. The elegant jar in the inset opposite, like the show globe, was an ornament pure and simple.

To promote patent medicines, manufacturers provided an astonishing variety of advertising signs, such as the plaster plaque below and the nearly life-sized statue—it is five feet high—of fisherman and cod *(right)* that was the trademark of a popular cod-liver-oil vitamin supplement. Occasionally a company went so far as to stage a live demonstration *(opposite)* of its product's purported powers.

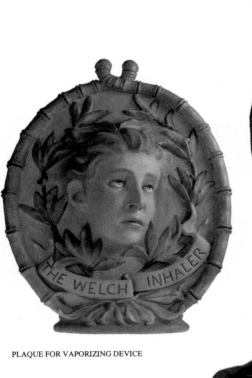

PLAQUE FOR VAPORIZING DEVICE

PAPIER-MÂCHÉ TRADEMARK OF SCOTT'S COD-LIVER OIL

Passersby draw close to a drugstore window as the piano-
playing marathon of a man named Mr. Taylor—he is described as
"a Specimen of Health, Strength and Vitality" —approaches
its 61st hour. The musician supposedly owed his stamina to
Digestit, a stomach aid whose promotional placards and
banners are filling the window of the store.

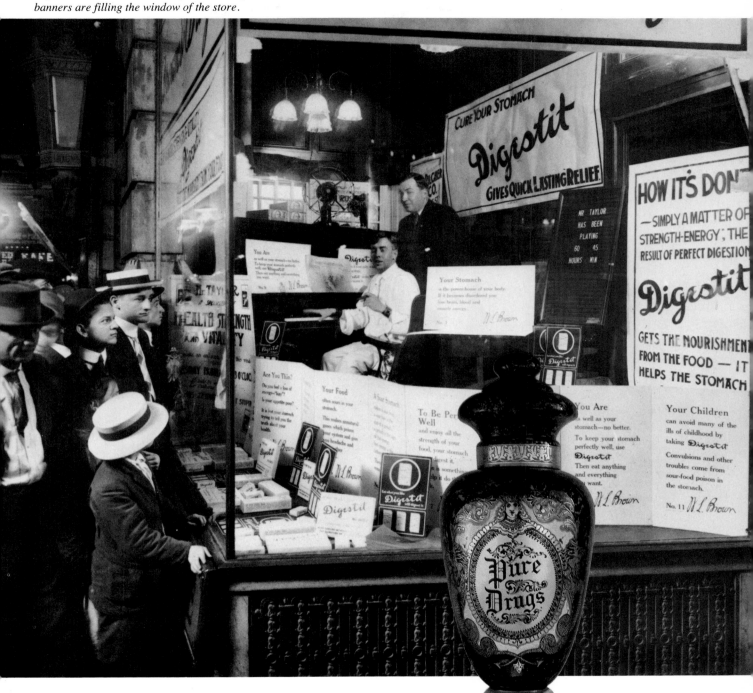

ORNAMENTAL JAR, USED FOR DISPLAY ONLY

Patrons of an Illinois pharmacy, photographed in 1902, gather around the store's central "island case"—filled with perfumed soaps on the upper shelf, scented oils and lotions on the lower. In the left foreground is the cigar and tobacco department.

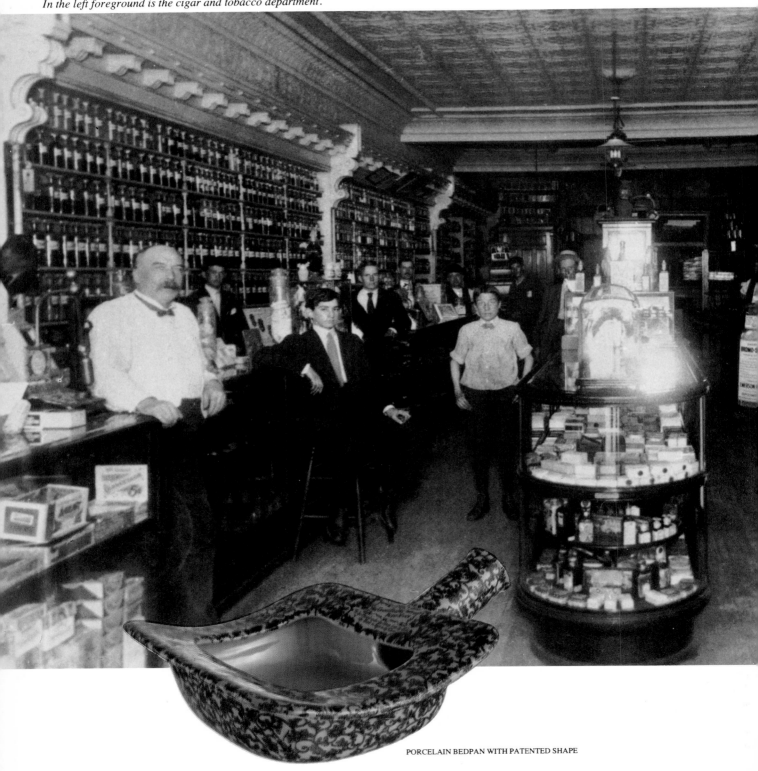

PORCELAIN BEDPAN WITH PATENTED SHAPE

A cornucopia of "sundries and fancy goods"

The "front of the store" in the old-fashioned pharmacy was the emporium that might offer for sale anything from paint to fertilizer. The listing of "sundries and fancy goods" in a drug wholesaler's catalogue of 1885 ran 200 pages—more than twice the space allotted to drugs. Included in the offerings were baskets of wire or willow, violin strings, backscratchers and assorted leather saddlebags.

Most of the items, however, had long been part of the traditional, if diversified, trade of the druggist. Some were medical equipment, others were nonprescription remedies such as leeches, stored alive in decorative ventilated jars *(right)* and sold for ancient bloodletting treatments. But many were nonmedicinal. "The perfume counter was the first one on the right as you entered the store," wrote Richard Armour of his father's California establishment. The perfumes, he remembered, were directly opposite another typical but nonmedicinal display—the cigar counter.

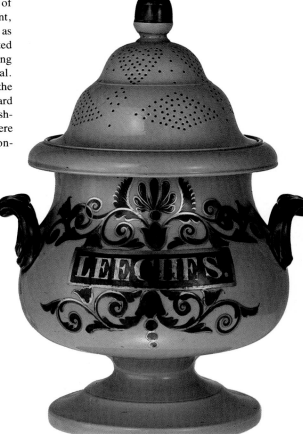

VENTILATED JAR FOR STORING 50 TO 75 LIVE LEECHES

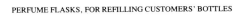

PERFUME FLASKS, FOR REFILLING CUSTOMERS' BOTTLES

Alchemy behind the counter

The pharmacist of 1900 had to be a short-order chemist, capable of creating at a moment's notice any medicine that a physician might prescribe. He did much more than count out pills; he employed a variety of devices to compound them from hundreds of chemicals and herbs kept in bottles, many of them elaborately decorated.

Precise measures of dry materials were weighed on a balance *(right, middle)* against coinlike weights in measures called drams (.0625 ounce) and scruples (.0208 ounce) used by apothecaries since classical times. To make spherical pills from the measured compounds, the druggist customarily pounded a slightly moistened mixture with a mortar and pestle. Then he placed the pasty blend in a pill machine *(right, bottom)*. When the machine's two sets of sharp, grooved blades bit through the compound, uniform pills were made.

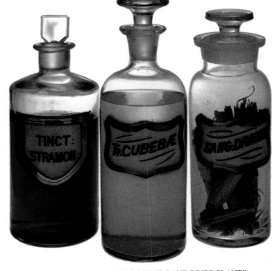

DISPENSING BOTTLES FOR LIQUIDS AND DRIED PLANTS

SPIKED BOTTLE FOR POISONS

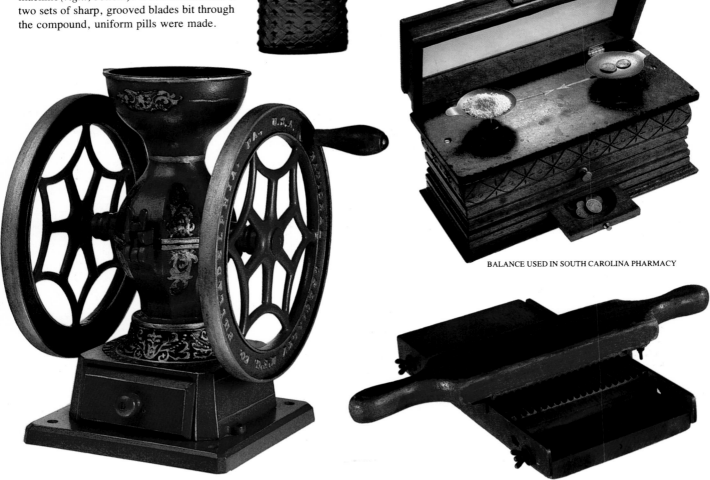

BALANCE USED IN SOUTH CAROLINA PHARMACY

CAST-IRON GRINDING MILL

BRASS-AND-WOOD PILL MACHINE, PATENTED 1872

*Three pharmacists compound medicines behind the
prescription counter of a Chicago drugstore in 1904. Only
a large city store was likely to employ a three-man staff to fill
prescriptions, or to decorate its drug counter with
an ornate wall frieze of garland-bearing cupids.*

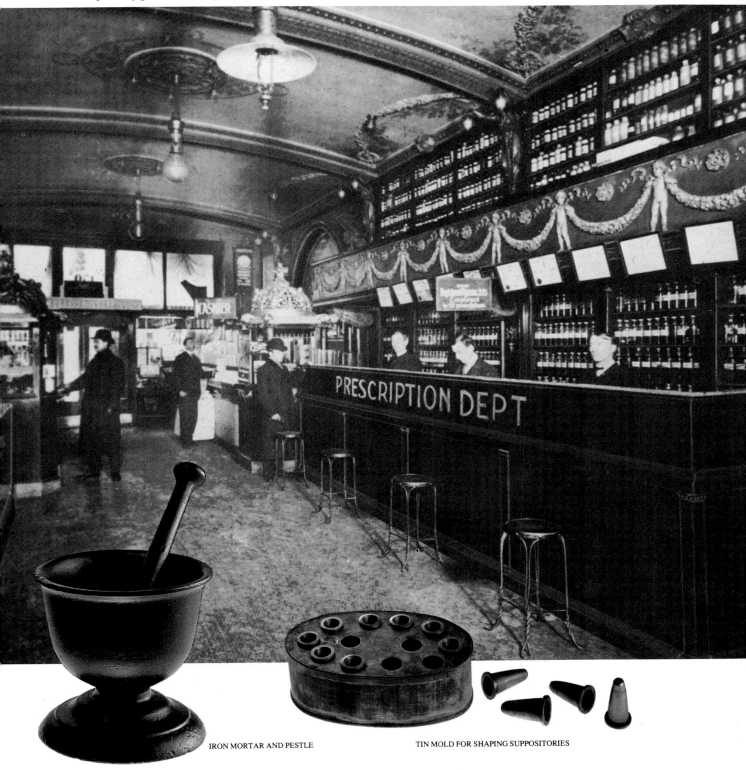

IRON MORTAR AND PESTLE   TIN MOLD FOR SHAPING SUPPOSITORIES

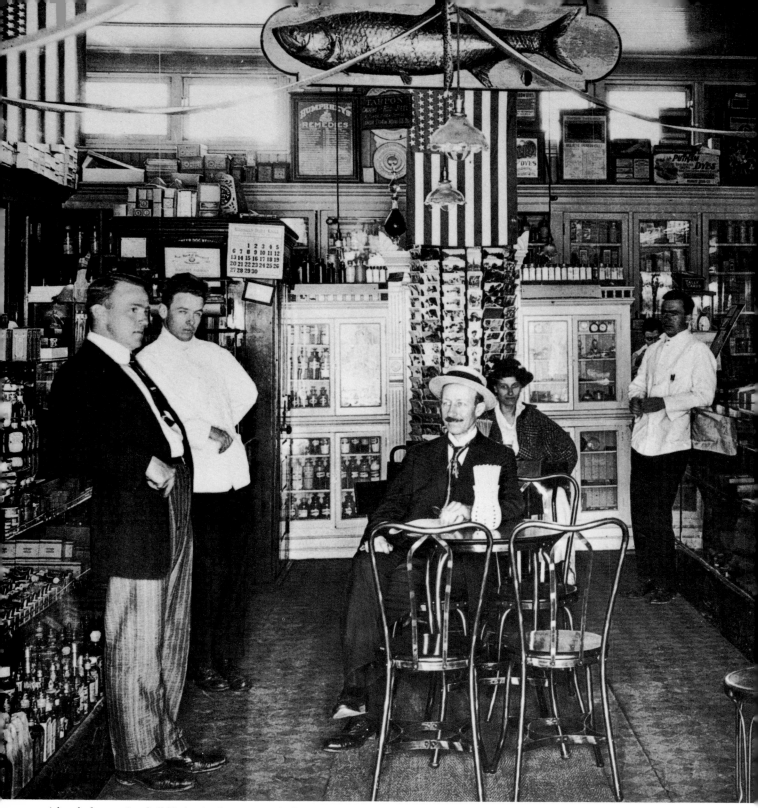

A locale for gossip of all kinds, the drugstore soda fountain dispensed proper—i.e., nonalcoholic—refreshments from its marble counter and gleaming nickel-plated fixtures. Some drinks were so famous they warranted special dispensers: Hires Root Beer from the barrel next to the white-jacketed soda jerk, Coca-Cola from the ornate jar (inset) at far right.

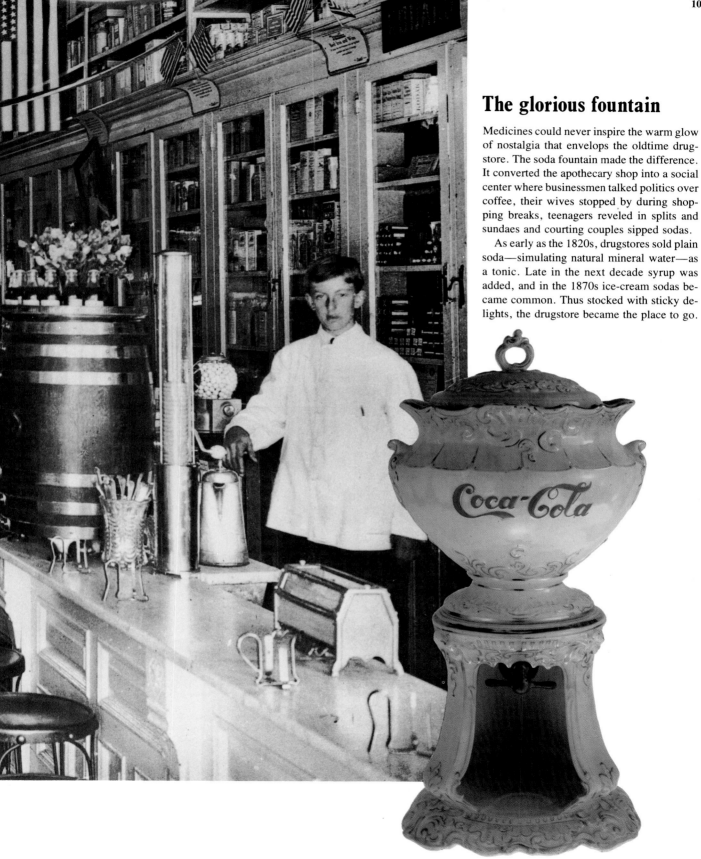

The glorious fountain

Medicines could never inspire the warm glow of nostalgia that envelops the oldtime drugstore. The soda fountain made the difference. It converted the apothecary shop into a social center where businessmen talked politics over coffee, their wives stopped by during shopping breaks, teenagers reveled in splits and sundaes and courting couples sipped sodas.

As early as the 1820s, drugstores sold plain soda—simulating natural mineral water—as a tonic. Late in the next decade syrup was added, and in the 1870s ice-cream sodas became common. Thus stocked with sticky delights, the drugstore became the place to go.

1896 SYRUP DISPENSER

CHAPTER 5

Working with the pharmacist

From pill peddlers to skilled professionals
An expert guide to drugs and their dangers
Picking generic products for savings
How to find the right pharmacist
Druggist of the future

You can buy medicines almost anywhere, in corner drugstores and chain outlets, supermarkets, discount houses and department stores, airports and hotels, even gas stations. Some places sell prescription drugs; others do not, and the difference is important. Those with prescription drugs contain an invaluable resource: a pharmacist, who can help you get the most effective use out of any medicine you buy.

Pharmacists can clarify a doctor's instructions for using a medicine or cut through the fog of advertising claims for competing over-the-counter products. They can save you money, by determining whether a brand-name product has a lower-cost counterpart. Most important, they can guard you against misused, misunderstood or misprescribed medicines.

Few of these highly trained specialists are known outside the communities they serve; some, particularly in the biggest and busiest stores, are faceless, anonymous figures even to their own customers. Yet every one of them stands in a unique position to protect medicine users against the dangers in drugs. Consider the following examples, all true, taken from scores of interviews conducted for this book.

● Pharmacist Dan Thomas of Irving, Texas, once refused to sell a cough remedy to a diabetic patient, explaining that the sweetened syrup could disrupt the blood-sugar balance involved in her diabetes. The woman walked out, bought the medicine at a grocery store—and wound up in the hospital.

● In California, Max Stollman protested when a Beverly Hills dentist prescribed cephalexin, an antibiotic chemically related to penicillin, for a patient allergic to penicillin. Stoll-

man warned that an allergy to one drug suggested an allergy to the other, but both patient and prescriber insisted he fill the order. The patient took the cephalexin and broke out in hives—an early sign of a potentially dangerous drug allergy.

● Barry Paraizo of West Palm Beach, Florida, received a prescription at his pharmacy for an unusually high dosage of a diuretic. Knowing that an overdose of the drug can cause such side effects as gout, Paraizo called the doctor and found that he had meant to prescribe a blood-pressure drug often used together with the diuretic. "His mind was thinking one thing, the old pen writing another," said Paraizo.

Every week more than 200 million people patronize the nation's 50,000 or so pharmacies, placing Thomas, Stollman, Paraizo and their colleagues at the cutting edge of professional counsel on the use of medicines, on side effects and on potential drug allergies and interactions. "My main job as a pharmacist," Stollman said, "is to help people be sensible medicine users." The job goes beyond processing prescriptions to the harder task of dispensing knowledge—knowledge that can benefit the public in unexpected ways. Some pharmacists routinely take readings of blood pressure, screen potential diabetics and provide emergency medical care. Others are experts in such specialized areas as geriatric medicine, cancer chemotherapy, and psychiatric drugs.

Hardly anyone who walks into a drugstore needs all the multiple services that pharmacists are now able to provide. But anyone who buys so much as a packet of aspirin can take advantage of a pharmacist's training and expertise. As dis-

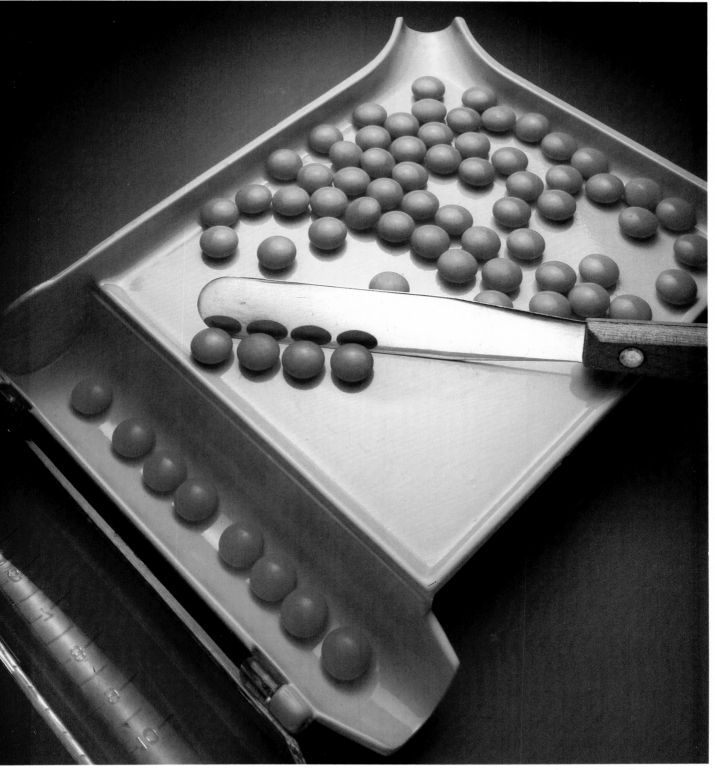

To guarantee against contamination, a pharmacist uses a spatula to push tablets into the trough of a tray (above); then he closes the cover, returns excess tablets to a stock container through the funnel (upper right), and empties the trough into a bottle. Such care protects not only the patient but also the pharmacist, who may react to contact with strong medicines.

pensers of both drugs and drug information, pharmacists are playing an ever more prominent part in caring for the health of Americans.

From pill peddler to skilled professional

In some ways this expanding role marks a return to a time-honored tradition. During the 1700s, the roles of pharmacists and physicians were often indistinguishable. General practitioners who served the remote American colonies styled themselves ''surgeon-apothecaries'' or ''dispensing physicians.'' They traveled from town to town with pills and potions that, more often than not, they had concocted. The luggage of these ''recipe doctors,'' reported the Medical Society of New Jersey in 1869, was ''pregnant with a promiscuous collection of remedies, concisely labeled 'Good for Rheumatism,' 'Good for the Piles,' 'Good for Fever and Ague.' '' The favorite prescriptions of Dr. John C. Budd, who plied his trade in the late 1700s around Camden, New Jersey, included an herbal brew he called ''Tincture Botanae''; he used it, he confided, when he did ''not know what else to do, for it was sedative, cathartic, tonic and expectorant, and cannot fail to hit somewhere.'' The uses of his other pet remedy—called ''Diabolical Pills''—are unknown.

These itinerant healers charged fees for consultations and surgery, but much of their income came from the medicines they sold. The prices ranged from one shilling—then enough to buy a pound of sugar—for a dose of ''alternative powder'' (said to alter the bodily ''humours,'' in Hippocrates' ancient theory of therapy) to seven shillings or more for decoctions containing such exotic substances as Peruvian bark, a crude form of quinine that did help victims of malaria.

As cities grew and medical entrepreneurs settled down, many carried on the pill-peddling tradition in dispensaries or apothecary shops adjoining their consulting chambers. Dispensaries operated by physicians were often called doctors' shops. Some others, run by men with no qualifications beyond a bit of scientific knowledge and a knack for trade, sold not only remedies but a host of other goods, from buttons to wagon wheels. In 1761 Benedict Arnold, later the prime villain of the American Revolution, set up shop in New Haven, Connecticut, as a ''Druggist, Bookseller &c. from London.'' Benjamin Franklin included in his own list of notable professions that of pharmacist; to supplement the income from his printing shop he opened a general store, where he sold such patent medicines as ''seneca rattlesnake root, with directions how to use it in pleurisy.''

In the 1800s the all-purpose practitioner began to disappear. The increasing complexity of medicine and the growing demands on physicians' time led most doctors to leave the selling of medicines to apothecaries, who compounded or selected drugs according to a doctor's written orders, or prescriptions. The profession of pharmacy emerged in turn; in 1821 the first American educational institution devoted to the field, the Philadelphia College of Pharmacy, opened its doors. But 19th Century pharmacists found that specialization did not pay the rent; most stocked their shops not only with drugs, but with nonmedicinal items as well.

By the early 20th Century the American drugstore had become a hub of community life. It was a place where people could get a headache powder, relax at the soda fountain, buy hairpins or candy, chat with neighbors, and perhaps get some medical advice from the friendly proprietor.

The drugstore owned by broadcaster Walter Cronkite's grandfather in Leavenworth, Kansas, was typical. ''It was a wondrous place,'' Cronkite recalled. ''Ruby urns cast a light that was full of warmth and mystery; high metal chairs stood before a marble refreshment counter, glass shelves held an endless assortment of pomades and nostrums. Aromatic smells filled the room. They came from the pharmacy in the rear, which contained row upon row of powders and liquids, a mortar and pestle, and a set of delicate scales. The bottles and boxes bore strange Latin names. Surely the man who presided over all this must be extraordinarily wise. And so my grandfather seemed to me.''

Much of the mystique and professional standing of such a pharmacist came from the fact that he put most of the medicines together himself. Until the early decades of the 20th Century, some 80 per cent of all prescriptions required a skilled pharmacist to compound the preparations from a variety of ingredients—including herbs he might have grown in his backyard. But with the rise of the modern pharmaceutical industry in the 1930s, more and more drugs were manufactured on assembly lines and shipped, ready to dispense. By the mid-1940s only a fourth of all prescriptions called for compounding by a pharmacist; by the late '70s the figure had dropped to less than 1 per cent.

An expert guide to drugs and their dangers

When giant pharmaceutical houses became the primary compounders of medicines, some of the pharmacist's traditional skills passed into obsolescence. But the central job of the profession remains the same: to stock the community medicine chest, to store the drugs safely, and to dispense these drugs uncontaminated and at full potency.

The job requires special schooling and is subject to governmental controls. Most U.S. pharmacists are trained in one of the nation's 72 accredited schools of pharmacy. To get a license to practice, the graduate must pass an examination by a state pharmacy board. To keep the license, he (or she: by the 1980s one out of every five licensed pharmacists and 50 per cent of all pharmacy students were women) must, in many states, take continuing-education courses.

Once in practice, a pharmacist continues to be regulated by the state board. The board sends inspectors unannounced to his pharmacy to examine storage conditions, spot-check for out-of-date drugs and scrutinize records and files. State record-keeping laws vary, but all require that prescriptions be kept on file for several years. In fact, according to Richard Penna, Director of Professional Affairs for the American Pharmaceutical Association (APA), "most pharmacists never get rid of their prescriptions. If you look in an older pharmacy's files, you can find those that date back decades."

One purpose of state inspection is to ensure compliance with federal laws on the sale of dangerous drugs such as narcotics. The law classifies "controlled substances" in five categories, called schedules, in decreasing order of potency and danger. No community pharmacy keeps the illegal substances of Schedule I, which includes heroin and LSD; few keep much in the way of Schedule II drugs such as morphine and cocaine, though these might be found in an area where

nursing homes use them to treat terminal cancer patients. Most pharmacies have a good supply of the frequently prescribed Schedule III and IV drugs—examples are acetaminophen with codeine (Schedule III) and the tranquilizer diazepam (Schedule IV); almost all stock the mild Schedule V items, such as cough syrups with small amounts of codeine.

By law, pharmacists must keep track of every controlled substance stocked. All prescriptions for them must be marked so that inspectors can check against the inventory. In some states Schedule V drugs can be dispensed without a prescription, but even they are kept behind the counter and customers must sign a log for each purchase.

The unsupervised inventories for other drugs vary widely. Most pharmacies stock several hundred commonly prescribed drugs; choices among the thousands of others on the market may depend on location. In a coal-mining area, for example, a pharmacy might carry a broad range of drugs for chronic lung diseases; in a suburb, pediatric drugs; in a retirement community, medicines for high blood pressure. But the stock also depends on the quirks of local physicians. "We've got one doctor in town who calls for one particular brand almost every time he wants a diuretic," said a West Virginia pharmacist. "Few doctors here prescribe it, but it's his favorite diuretic, so we always keep a few bottles of it around."

Actually, most pharmacies do not stock huge quantities of any single prescription drug. For most medicines, there will be a large bottle containing up to a thousand tablets or capsules or a gallon of liquid. Prepackaged drugs, such as ointments, may be represented by only a few individual doses. But pharmacies can generally obtain any missing drugs quite quickly. In large cities and suburbs, drug wholesalers deliver most orders the day they are placed; in small communities or rural areas, they deliver within 24 hours.

Because most medicines arrive ready to dispense, the pharmacist's traditional tools—mortar and pestle, scales, funnels and the like—are rarely needed. Considering the pace of a modern pharmacy's trade, that is probably all to the good. Prescriptions often come across the counter like a blizzard, some 150 to 200 a day in a busy store. For each one, the pharmacist need only get the medicine, select a container and pour in the medicine or count out the required pills.

As most customers suspect, there is no great trick to counting out tablets. Some pharmacists use special counting devices *(page 103);* others pour tablets onto sheets of paper and count by eye. The advantage of paper is that it is disposable; after a pharmacist counts out a drug such as penicillin, which leaves a faint, powdery residue that can contaminate another prescription, the paper is discarded. According to Richard Penna of the APA, patients are not the only ones who risk contamination. One of the pharmacist's few occupational hazards is a sensitivity to penicillin; some become so allergic to the drug that they have to leave the profession.

After measuring out a drug, the pharmacist types a prescription label bearing the patient's and physician's name, the date, the name of the drug and a translation of the doctor's cryptic instructions *(page 62)* on dosage and use. In some states, the pharmacist must include the drug's expiration date. He then stamps both the prescription and the label with the number under which the prescription will be filed, and pastes the label to the container. Finally, he may add a few supplementary labels: warnings to "Shake well before using," "Use special care when operating a car," and the like.

Good pharmacists do not stop there. Some states require pharmacists to hand over each prescription personally and discuss it with the patient. Even without the compulsion of law, many pharmacists make it a point to explain prescriptions. And they often call doctors before filling one. They may point out conflicting drugs prescribed by different specialists or report suspicious indications of drug abuse—for example, a patient who brings in a number of prescriptions from different doctors for a potent tranquilizer. At times they catch grim examples of physician carelessness, such as an adult dosage prescribed for a child.

The protection a pharmacist can give extends to nonprescription products. Most pharmacists regard them with caution. Max Stollman said, "I keep all of my medicines in the back of the counter, so that people will have to ask for them and I can say, 'Why are you taking this?' or, 'You have to be careful when you drive a car if you're on this.' "

A pharmacist who knows his customers and watches over their purchases can often save them from harm. He might warn a customer with ulcers not to buy aspirin because it irritates the lining of the stomach, or caution a glaucoma sufferer that a popular cold remedy contains belladonna, which can increase pressure within the eye. Dan Thomas recalled the day a couple came into his pharmacy to buy a nonprescription medicine for their daughter. "She was about five or six years old and she had real puffy eyes, swollen to the point where they were almost closed." Thomas gave the child's leg a gentle prod. "She had pitting edema."

Pitting edema, a puffy swelling that leaves a small depression when the skin is pressed, is often a symptom of heart or kidney disease. Thomas told the girl's parents to get her to a doctor. "To try an over-the-counter medicine on her is like trying to treat leprosy with aspirin. They could have bought all the stuff over the counter they wanted for this child, but the child would have developed further problems and probably within two or three years would be dead. When people like that come in, I won't sell them anything."

Picking generic products for savings

Not only can a pharmacist use his medical expertise to save a life, but he can save his customers money. He knows how to pick the best drugs at the most reasonable prices. Usually, that means picking a drug by the generic name of its active ingredient rather than by a brand name given by a manufacturer. A drug's brand name is invariably shorter, simpler and easier to remember than its generic name. It was designed to be so. A generic name is generally an abbreviated version of a long, often heroically complex chemical description. The full chemical name of a certain antihistamine, for example, is Ethanamine,2-(diphenylmethoxy)-N,N-dimethyl,-HCL. The full generic name is diphenhydramine hydrochloride. It is generally shortened further to diphenhydramine, but even so, to the patients who take it—and to many physicians who prescribe it—it will always be known as Benadryl, the trade name given by the developer.

About half of the most commonly prescribed drugs—including Benadryl—and most nonprescription drugs are sold under many different brand names. Although the active

From open-air bazaar to prescription palace

During the early Middle Ages, Western science and medicine were in the capable hands of the Moslems, who dominated much of the Mediterranean world. In the Eighth Century they established in Baghdad the first privately owned stores that dealt mainly in medicines: the direct ancestors of the modern drugstore. In a book from that period, physician Ibn 'Abd Rabbih described these small open-air stands as offering their customers "all useful medications that could be manufactured: syrups, essences and conserves, electuaries, confections, sternutatories, eye salves, oily extracts, and all types of medicated powders, spiced perfumes, and cosmetics."

The varied stock of the pharmacy—including not only drugs but also sweets and cosmetics—was thus established as a tradition. Only the store changed. The Moslem conquest of Spain and Sicily, followed by the Crusades and the Renaissance, brought Arab-style pharmacies to Europe. By the end of the 16th Century many were sheltered from the street, sometimes behind glass windows.

By the 18th Century, the European pharmacy, flourishing under the patronage of princes and the control of guilds, displayed shelves laden with ceramic drug jars in an elaborate dispensing room, while out of sight in a back room was a compounding area—an arrangement still seen today.

An early Arab pharmacy, depicted in a 13th Century Turkish painting, opened directly onto busy city streets. The druggist stored his wares, including thousands of drugs, in hanging leather bags and in tin-glazed earthenware jars.

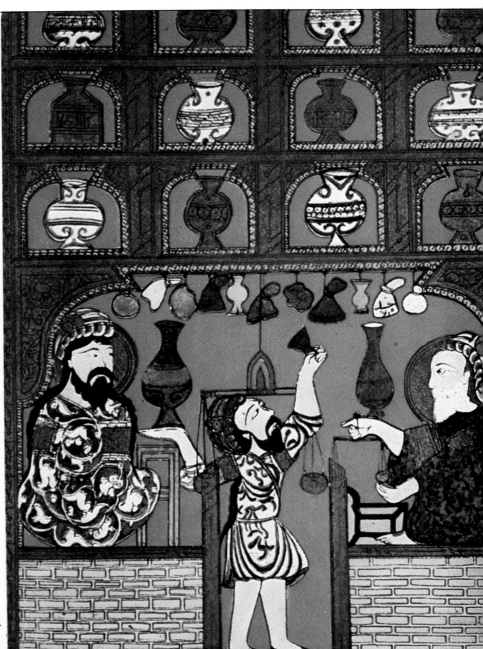

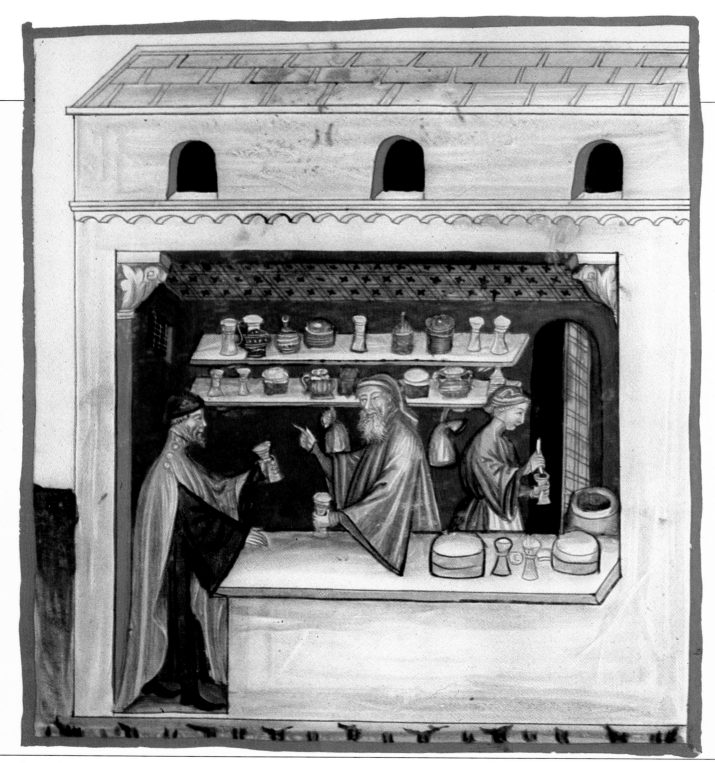

In a 14th Century Italian pharmacy, little changed from the Arab original, a druggist dispenses theriac, a potion concocted from more than 100 ingredients and used for centuries in Europe as a poison antidote and cure-all. The front counter folded up at night to help protect the expensive drugs from thieves.

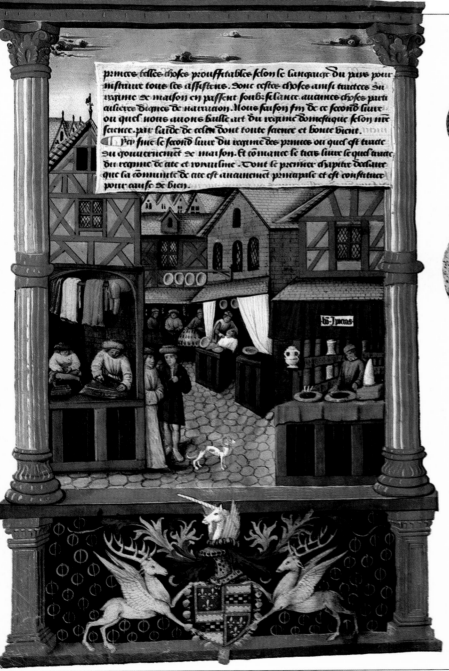

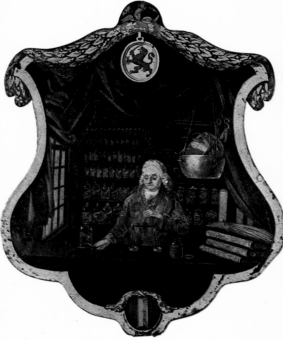

The shield of a 17th Century pharmacists' guild in the Netherlands bears a picture of the druggist at work. He prepares a prescription with the aid of a hand scale and three large books, possibly pharmacopeias that list the formulas of various medicines. The shield also has the guild insignia: a lion (top) and a bar (bottom).

A French apothecary shop (right foreground) opens onto a narrow cobblestone street in a drawing from an early-16th Century manuscript. Displayed prominently on the druggist's front counter is a cone of sugar, which, like the spiced wine advertised in the inscription at top, was also sold there.

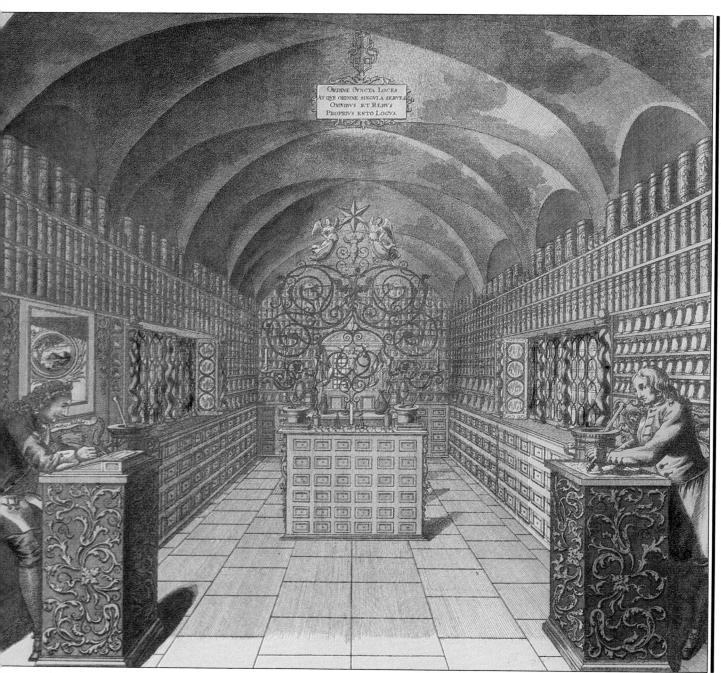

ORDINE CVNCTA LOCES
ATQVE ORDINE SINGVLA SERVES
OMNIBVS ET REBVS
PROPRIVS ESTO LOCVS.

The Pharmacy of the Golden Star in Nuremberg, pictured in an 18th Century engraving, resembles an ornate version of the modern drugstore. A physician (left) records a prescription while the pharmacist prepares a dispensing container. The grillwork over the counter in the center separates the front dispensing area from the compounding laboratory in the rear.

ingredients in the various brands are identical, the prices are not. The most familiar example is aspirin—the generic name for acetylsalicylic acid—which is sold in hundreds of brands, some four times more expensive than others.

Less well known is the potential economy in ordering prescription drugs by generic chemical composition rather than by brand name. At a time when 24 capsules of the diarrhea remedy Lomotil retailed for $6.24, the same drug was being sold under its generic name, diphenoxylate, for $3.85 per 24 tablets—a 38.3 per cent savings. Because Lomotil and diphenoxylate are two names for the same drug, it made obvious economic sense to buy the cheaper version.

Less obviously, it might not have made medical sense. Whether you ought to take advantage of such a savings depends on considerations not covered by the drug label. Ever since the economics of purchasing drugs by generic name first came to public attention, the wisdom of doing so has been debated. The controversy, carried on by physicians, pharmacists and pharmacologists, hinges on the question of whether two medicines with the same active ingredients but from different sources have exactly the same therapeutic effect—in the language of pharmacology, whether they have therapeutic bioequivalence. Some do, and some do not.

A pharmacist can help you decide when buying a generic drug is a worthwhile economy, because he understands the technical and business practices that cause differences in price. Some brands of drugs cost more than others simply because their makers spend a lot of money advertising and distributing them. This influence on price applies to a few prescription drugs as well as to nonprescription medicines, many of which are available both as costly advertised brands and as low-priced, little-known brands.

Manufacturing methods also affect price; some drugs may be so cheaply made that their reliability and effectiveness are impaired by variations in density or concentration, in the quality of inactive ingredients and even in the proportions of active ingredients. Finally, laws regulating development, testing and patenting of new drugs *(Chapter 6)* have a great impact on price: Drugs awarded U.S. patents are more costly while the patent remains in force, but become available in cheaper brands after the patent expires. When a new drug—a unique chemical with a specific therapeutic effect—is patented, its developer receives exclusive marketing rights for 17 years. Thus, most new drugs enter the market with a premium price tag.

They also enter the world with a registered brand or trade name, used to promote the drug. After a drug goes off patent, the company that developed it retains sole rights to the original brand name; competing manufacturers that duplicate the drug sell it under its generic name or register a trade name of their own. Relatively unburdened by heavy research and promotion expenses, these manufacturers produce the drug at lower cost and sell it at a correspondingly lower price.

Because of the price difference, government health agencies, the military and other large-scale purchasers of drugs make it a general practice to buy and dispense generic drugs; the major exceptions to the rule are drugs still under patent and therefore available solely as brand-name products. In many hospitals, all prescribing is done generically unless a doctor insists on a particular brand. Many physicians in private practice habitually prescribe by brand name. The practice is changing—slowly. In 1970 only 7 per cent of the prescriptions written by private physicians were for generic drugs; a decade later, the percentage had doubled. But the fact remains that more than six out of every seven prescriptions written in the United States are for brand names.

One reason so few prescriptions are written generically is that, unlike pharmacists, many doctors have only a hazy notion of how much medicines actually cost. In 1978, less than a third of the 114 doctors responding to a survey of the Philadelphia area could guess to within 20 per cent the prices of the drugs they most commonly prescribed. Another explanation of doctors' preference for brand names is simple enough. As the respected Washington, D.C., cardiologist Michael Halberstam once admitted: "Sometimes I prescribe by brand name because I don't remember the generic name."

Doctors remember the brand name partly because it is heavily promoted during the patent period. Advertisements in medical publications and periodic visits from drug company representatives called detail men make certain the product and its virtues are known. After the patent expires, many doctors continue to write the familiar brand name in prescriptions, partly because it is familiar but also for more important reasons: They have had experience with the drug that bears the name they trust and sometimes they have reservations about the quality and efficacy of competing products.

In some cases their caution is justified. Many factors influence bioavailability—the rate and extent of a drug's absorption into the body—which determines whether or not the drug is therapeutically equivalent to other drugs in its generic class. During the manufacturing process, such inert ingredients as bindings, fillers, flavorings, colorings, coatings and preservatives are added to a drug. All can affect its bioavailability. But unlike the active components of a drug, inactive ones are a trade secret—information on them is supplied to the Food and Drug Administration, but not to the public.

Other differences in a drug's absorption in the body can arise from the mechanics of production. Even the degree of pressure in a machine that stamps out tablets can affect a drug's efficacy: The more tightly a tablet is compressed, the more slowly it will dissolve. Atlanta physician Mark Zimmerman, a pharmacy school graduate as well as a doctor, made that point about a drug as simple as aspirin. "Take 10 different brands of aspirin and throw them against a wall," he suggested, "A couple will crumble, but the rest will bounce all over the room. They have the same amount of aspirin, but some are packed so tightly that they could pass through the digestive tract without dissolving." Though the mechanics of manufacturing drugs have improved, Dr. Zimmerman warns that wide variations in bioavailability exist.

In particularly potent drugs, such differences in bioavailability are crucial. For example, there is only a slim margin of safety between therapeutic and lethal doses of the heart stimulant digoxin and the antiepilepsy drug phenytoin. Physicians tend to play it safe when prescribing such drugs, putting their faith in brand-name products, trusting the quality control and testing procedures of an original manufacturer or a famous pharmaceutical house to protect their patients from subpotent or superpotent drugs.

Surprisingly often, however, their faith may be misplaced.

It is not only impossible to judge the quality of a drug by its manufacturer, but it can be difficult to find out the manufacturer. A medicine that bears the name of a major pharmaceutical company may never have seen that company's factory; conversely, some drugs sold under generic names have what are thought of as distinguished origins. About 90 per cent of all generic drugs are distributed by the same companies that develop the brand-name drugs: The giant Eli Lilly and Company is one of the nation's largest manufacturers of generic drugs. Many large firms produce entire lines of so-called branded generics, with names that may combine trade and generic terms; one example is SK-Ampicillin, produced by the well-known Smith Kline and French Company.

These large companies may distribute but not actually manufacture their own generics. According to a report issued by the New York State Assembly in 1978, Lederle Laboratories distributed approximately 83 generics—all but "possibly" two of which, the report said, were manufactured by other companies, large and small. Lederle's version of the tranquilizer chlordiazepoxide, for example, was made by a company named Barr Laboratories. It sold to pharmacists under the Lederle name at $17.01 for 500 capsules. Barr supplied the same drug to the Darby Drug Company, which sold the same quantity for $4.85. In an even more extreme case, three major pharmaceutical houses sold an antibiotic, erythromycin stearate, as a generic. The tablets came in different colors and shapes and were sold at different prices. But all were manufactured in a single plant in Morgantown, West Virginia, by a company named Mylan Laboratories.

To add to the irony, large research firms with patents on some brand-name drugs often contract with other companies to make them. Thus, few physicians prescribing those brands know whether the medicine a patient gets came from the originator's own factory or some other firm's.

Pharmacists, on the other hand, generally do know or can find out. The nature of their job gives them first-hand knowledge of the substandard or questionable drugs that occasionally do reach the market. Sometimes the evidence is right in front of their eyes: tablets that disintegrate in the bottle or are so hard they may not dissolve at all, preparations whose

Pharmacists who made their mark

In Benjamin Franklin, a knowledge of pharmacy occasionally inspired a certain cynicism. ''He's the best physician that knows the worthlessness of the most medicines,'' Franklin once wrote. Yet medicinal drugs remained a strong interest of the polymath Founding Father, and when he helped establish Pennsylvania Hospital in 1751, he created America's first hospital apothecary, to ''make up Medicines only, according to the Prescriptions.''

Franklin was only one of many people famous for achievements outside medicine who served as pharmacists. Isaac Newton developed his preoccupation with science—as well as lifelong hypo-chondria—while helping an apothecary as a boy. The Norwegian dramatist Henrik Ibsen wrote his first play while employed in a rural apothecary shop. Before embarking on his infamous military career, Benedict Arnold ran a drugstore in Connecticut and delighted in being addressed as ''Dr. Arnold.''

O. Henry, the American short-story writer, drew on memories of his uncle's drugstore for many vivid characterizations. A licensed pharmacist, he worked as a prison druggist while in jail for embezzlement. And Hubert Humphrey, U.S. Senator for 23 years and Vice President, began his working life as a pharmacist.

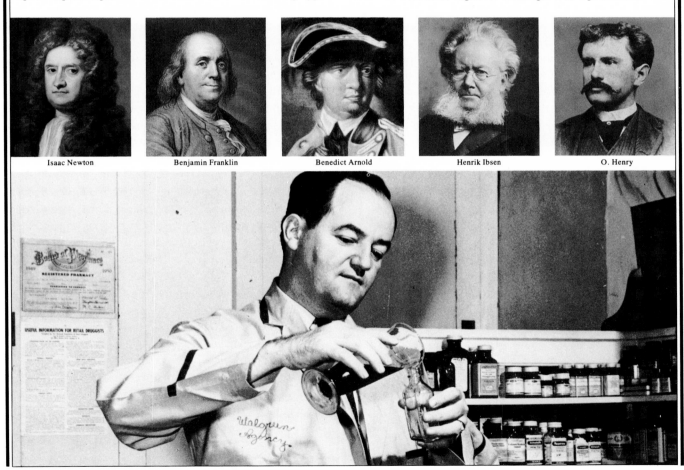

Isaac Newton   Benjamin Franklin   Benedict Arnold   Henrik Ibsen   O. Henry

Hubert Humphrey, taking time off from the United States Senate in 1949, helps out in his family's South Dakota drugstore, where he was a partner and licensed pharmacist. Humphrey often debated politics with customers. He met his future wife in the store, when she dropped by one day for a soda.

odor is off, or liquids contaminated by visible particles.

A pharmacist can also make accurate judgments on less obvious problems involving certain drugs' therapeutic effects, including the sometimes subtle differences in bioavailability. Both physicians and pharmacists have access to studies in professional journals, FDA reports and research data supplied by manufacturers. But a pharmacist's ability to evaluate that information equals or exceeds that of many doctors. His training in biopharmaceutics—the study of a drug's formulation and its activity within the body—is far more extensive than that of most physicians. In the late 1970s medical students at the University of Missouri attended one to three lectures on drug actions during their course of studies; the typical pharmacy student attended 30 to 60.

According to Richard Penna, pharmacists are more discriminating and skeptical about manufacturer-supplied data. They can look at a chemical structure, or even a name (because generic names reveal something about biological and chemical characteristics) and make certain inferences—how a new drug compares to one already on the market, for example, or whether a so-called improved formula does in fact offer a genuine improvement in theraputic effect.

Increasingly, pharmacists have legal authority to back up their knowledge. Most states have passed drug-product selection laws that place the burden of evaluating the relative merits of drugs on pharmacists. Generally, the laws allow a pharmacist to dispense a generic drug in place of the equivalent brand-name medicine unless the prescribing physician forbids it by writing ''medically necessary'' or ''dispense as written'' on the prescription form. In a few states pharmacists are required to dispense the cheaper drug whenever possible; in most, they must be asked to do so by the patient.

Such laws are modeled after the practices of many hospitals. In those where all prescribing is done generically, staff pharmacists and selection committees of physicians monitor drug purchases. Filling prescriptions is left to the judgment of the hospital pharmacist, working from the institution's list of acceptable choices, known as a formulary. Many states now have their own formularies—based on a list provided by the FDA—incorporated in their selection laws. So-called positive formularies are lists of drugs officially rated therapeutically equivalent within each generic category. Some states have negative formularies, also based on government data, listing drugs that are not appropriate substitutes.

How to find the right pharmacist

The problem for many consumers, perhaps, is finding a pharmacist who has the training and inclination to provide such expert, comprehensive guidance. Because medicines are so widely available, most people get them at a variety of sources. To get the full advantage of a pharmacist's services, you must choose a single pharmacy that meets your family's needs, then buy essentially all your medicines there.

Many considerations enter into the choice—convenience, prices, service reliability—but one that is very important yet often overlooked is the existence of an effective system to monitor all the drugs that your family may buy. Most pharmacies today keep some form of patient medication profiles, essential to safe and effective drug use. ''Don't go to a pharmacist who doesn't use them,'' is the blunt advice of Joe Forno, owner of a pharmacy in Woodstock, New York.

Patient profiles range from simple card files to elaborate computerized systems that retrieve existing data, enter a new prescription in the record and even type labels. But however primitive or sophisticated the record may be, both the APA and the Academy of Pharmacy Practice recommend that it contain the following information:

● Your name, address and telephone number.

● Your date of birth, and those of other family members. This item is not an intrusion upon your privacy: It helps the pharmacist to check whether a specific drug or dosage is appropriate, given the user's age.

● Allergies, distinctive reactions or other adverse effects you have shown after taking a drug, and the names of any medicines that have proved ineffective for you.

● Health conditions or diseases such as diabetes, ulcers or high blood pressure that preclude the use of certain drugs.

● The nonprescription medicines you use regularly, such as painkillers, antacids, laxatives, antihistamines and vitamin or mineral supplements.

• The date and number of each prescription filled for you, the name of the drug, its dosage form and strength, the quantity dispensed, the directions for use and the price. This item should also include the name and address of the doctor and the initials of the pharmacist who filled the prescription.

Properly used by the pharmacist, the profiles can catch prescription mistakes, screen conflicting medicines and warn of unsuitable combinations of prescription and over-the-counter drugs. What is more, they can help prevent errors in medication on the part of the patient. If, for example, a patient orders a prescription refill prematurely, the pharmacist can determine whether the directions for its use have been misinterpreted—an error easily made when someone used to taking a medicine twice a day switches to an improved drug that need be taken only once a day. Finally, the profile pays a practical dividend: It provides a record for tax or insurance purposes of all expenditures for medicines.

Beyond the importance of a medication profile, there are a number of other practical considerations to bear in mind when you pick a pharmacy. Find out what days and hours it is open, and check to be sure that a pharmacist is on duty at all these times to give advice or fill an urgent prescription. Ask if a pharmacist is available for emergency calls after hours or on a Sunday or holiday. And find out whether the pharmacy will deliver a prescription to your home or office.

Most pharmacies honor government health insurance and similar insurance plans; if this is a factor in your decision, ask about it in advance. In any case, check the pharmacy's prices on prescription drugs. Several states now require pharmacies to post a selection of prescription prices. Whether your pharmacy does or not, you are entitled to ask what a particular medicine will cost before you have a prescription filled, and you should compare the price with those of other pharmacies for the same drug. To some extent, the price will depend on a pharmacy's basic pricing procedures.

Many pharmacies have replaced the traditioal percentage markup with a fixed dispensing or professional fee, added to each prescription regardless of the cost of the medicine. The flat fee has certain advantages: It puts the transaction on a professional basis, removing any incentive to give a custom-er a higher-priced form of a medicine when a lower-priced equivalent is available. On less expensive drugs, the fee may seem high—a three-dollar fee, for example, on a bottle of tablets that cost the pharmacist three dollars represents a 100 per cent markup—but it reflects the cost of the pharmacist's time and skills more accurately than a percentage rate. And the same three-dollar fee would be applied to a $15 prescription, which calls for the same time, expertise and effort.

Finally, if anyone in your family needs special health products in addition to medicines, look for a pharmacy that supplies or can get them. Many pharmacies stock a wide range of orthopedic equipment and employ certified fitters; others sell and can instruct patients in the use of prostheses. Some pharmacies have entire home health-care centers staffed by trained personnel, where a family can rent or purchase hospital equipment for a bedridden patient.

In the long run, a pharmacy is only as good as the pharmacist who practices there—something you cannot judge fully until you have used the pharmacy for a while. From the start, however, you can watch for some touchstones of good practice. A pharmacist should, at your request, tell you whether there is a therapeutically equivalent generic product available for the brand-name drug your doctor has prescribed. If you have a condition that will require taking quantities of a medicine over an extended period, he should tell you whether you can save any money and the time spent picking up refills by getting a larger-than-normal supply that will stay fresh at the rate you use it. If you have trouble opening child-resistant bottle caps, and there are no young children at home, he should provide the medication in a container with a conventional screw or cap top. Each time a prescription is filled, the pharmacist should check your record for potential problems. If he spots an inconsistency in prescribing, a suspect dosage or an unclear notation, he should do more than mention that fact; he should call the doctor involved and settle the matter.

Above all, he should patiently answer any questions you have about your medication. No pharmacist should ever be too busy to answer such questions. Barry Pearlman, who sees thousands of patients every year at a busy Cleveland store, put it this way: "I'm the family pharmacist. If someone has

A global variety of dispensing styles

Pharmacies outside the United States can be very different from the drugs-to-groceries emporiums familiar to Americans. Sometimes the drugs are familiar but the style is not: In the Soviet Union, for example, pharmacies sell medicines almost exclusively, and in urban areas, stores must maintain a laboratory for compounding drugs. Elsewhere the stock is mixed; in China, customers can choose ancient herbal or modern chemical medicines. In some African nations, such as Kenya, rural areas have no pharmacies; instead, clinical teams fly in to dispense drugs.

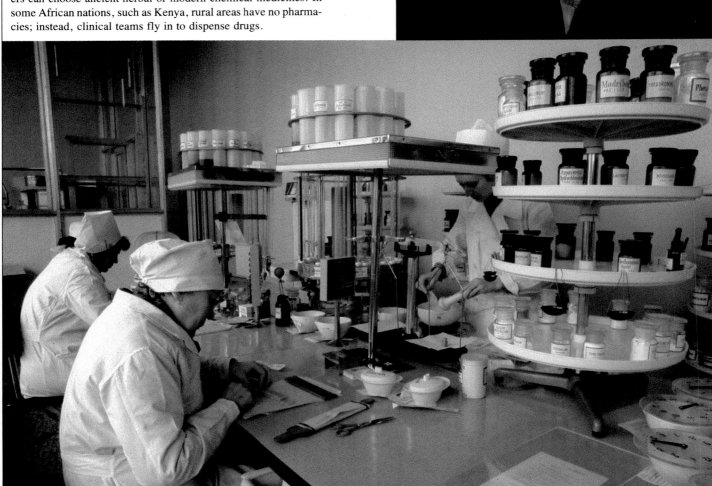

Wearing a surgical mask during the influenza season, a Moscow pharmacist (top) examines a prescription as two customers look on. In the adjoining laboratory (above), medicines are compounded by hand, with equipment ranging from the sophisticated timing clocks at lower right to the old-fashioned mortar and pestle in the background.

In the interior of Kenya, Masai women have prescriptions filled at a mobile health unit set up under a thorn tree. In this remote bush country, accessible to doctors and nurses only by airplane, even bottles are precious; patients must return empty drug containers to be sterilized and reused.

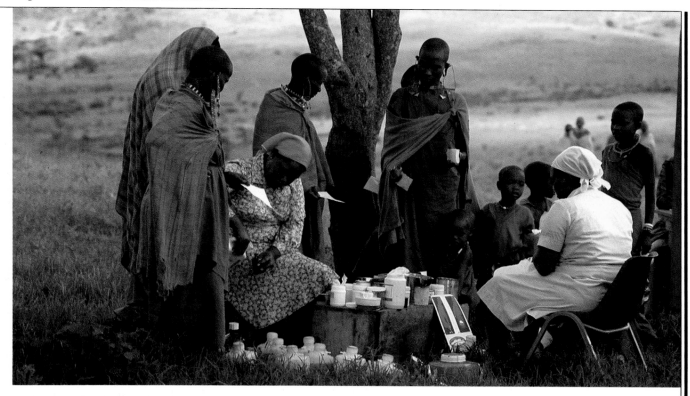

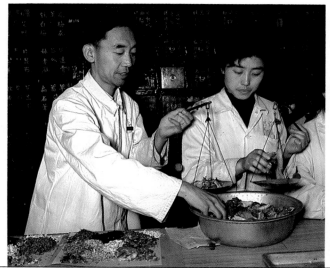

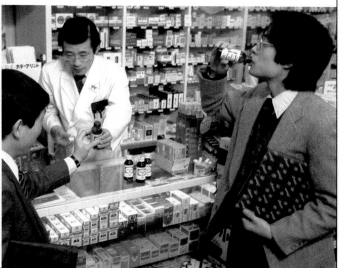

At Tang Ren Tang, a Peking pharmacy famous for its many herbal medicines, druggists weigh ingredients in hand scales; they will prepare the ingredients in the forms at lower left and mix them according to old formulas. Most Chinese pharmacies offer modern prescription drugs, but traditional remedies are so widely used that virtually every drugstore sells them.

In a well-stocked American-style drugstore in Tokyo, two hurried customers buy a patent medicine on their way to work and down it on the spot. The elixir—a mixture of B vitamins, ginseng, musk oil amd caffeine—is said to cure fatigue, headaches and hangovers. Japanese pharmacists are expected to dispense free medical advice along with medicines.

118

time for a question, I have time for answers.'' Do not accept less. The pharmacist's role in fostering the intelligent use of medicines and in guarding against improper use makes him as essential a member of your personal health-care team as your doctor and dentist.

Druggist of the future

Large as the role of pharmacists has become, it is almost certain to continue to grow. Their expanding responsibilities are indicated by the new drug-selection laws giving them wide discretion in filling prescriptions. Even their stores are changing. The soda fountain of fond memory is almost gone. Increasingly the trade in general merchandise and even non-prescription medicines is left to the supermarkets—which by 1978 had taken over 47 per cent of all nonprescription drug sales as more pharmacists focused their expertise on pre-

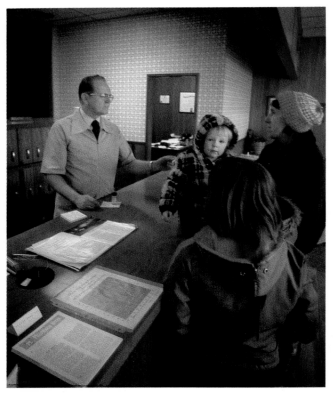

Pharmacist Eugene White hands dosage instructions to a patient who has brought her children to his unusual, office-style pharmacy in Berryville, Virginia. Uncluttered by conventional drug displays, greeting cards and sundries, White's pharmacy substitutes health-information literature and discreet wooden cabinets containing nonprescription drugs.

scriptions and other direct aids to the practicing physician.

The pharmacist's future role has been anticipated by professionals like Eugene White. In 1957, seven years out of the Medical College of Virginia School of Pharmacy, White was disillusioned by his job as a traditional druggist in a traditional drugstore. ''I wondered,'' he later recalled, ''why a pharmacist spent four years in school studying pharmacy just to come out and start selling paint and cutting glass and dispensing Cokes.'' He wondered, too, whether the proliferation of new drugs might point to a new role for the pharmacist. ''At that time we were seeing five to six hundred new drugs a year, and one day the thought crossed my mind that if I'm having trouble keeping up with pharmacy, how is a physician keeping up?'' White began to envisage a time when pharmacists would not just store and dispense a huge inventory of medicines, but would monitor their use and act as drug advisers to physicians and patients.

To put his new ideas into practice, White bought a drugstore in the little town of Berryville, Virginia. First he stripped it of its magazine racks. Then he told the bus company to find itself another terminal. Finally, he ripped out the soda fountain, cosmetic counter and greeting-card display, concealed his drugs behind wooden paneling and hung up a new sign: ''Eugene V. White, Pharmacist.'' The day he opened the doors, he recalled, ''People came in and said, 'Where's the drugstore?' And I said, 'This is the pharmacy office. And it is what a drugstore really should look like.' ''

Obviously, White's idea of a drugstore was not a store at all. It was a professional center, in which the counseling of patients and the monitoring of drug use took precedence over the dispensing of medicines. To that end, he developed one of the first medication-profile systems. He also set aside a private room in which he could take drug histories and discuss drug therapy with patients. ''This is where the pharmacist will be in the future,'' he says of his tiny consulting chamber, ''not standing in the midst of a giant emporium.''

White is an admitted visionary. He foresees the day when a pharmacist will prescribe medicines, at the stage after a doctor makes a diagnosis and before a technician counts out the pills. Already apparent is a shifting emphasis in pharmacy education from a technical proficiency with chemicals to the broader concepts of clinical care. Most American schools of pharmacy are now associated with teaching hospitals, bringing pharmacy students into close contact with other health-care professionals *(pages 120-133)*. Many schools offer advanced degrees in specialized fields of therapeutic work.

Armed with their new knowledge, pharmacists have begun to take on some functions once reserved to physicians. Thousands of pharmacists are now trained to take their customers' blood pressure readings, and refer them to a physician if necessary. In the future they may take on other duties such as diabetes screening, minor emergency medical treatment and immunization shots.

In some areas, the hospital-based working relationship between physician and pharmacist has been transferred to community settings. When Robert E. Davis was a graduate pharmacy student at the Medical University of South Carolina, he met Drs. William Crigler and Henry Martin, medical residents at the university's program for family practitioners. When the three completed their studies, they moved to Lexington, South Carolina, and went into practice together, sharing the same waiting room, business office and clinical resources. Later they were joined by two other physicians. When any of the four doctors in the building wrote a prescription—sometimes after consultation with Davis—the doctor sent the patient to the pharmacist, who took a drug history and checked for allergies, drug duplications or potential drug interactions. The pharmacist then discussed with the patient the proper use and possible side effects of the medicine.

"The first time they are sent to me, some of them say, 'This is a racket. Why do I need to talk to a pharmacist?' " Davis reported. "But then, most of them say, 'Hey, this is nice. I've never had this done before.' " And Davis added, "This is the only way I would practice pharmacy."

Some pharmacists practice pharmacy without ever dispensing a pill. Beatrice Adreon worked in a Washington, D.C., suburb as a pharmacy consultant for patients referred to her by area physicians, pharmacies, nursing homes and retirement centers. After taking a personal and medical history, she instructed patients about the purposes and use of both their prescription and nonprescription medicines and advised physicians about possible alterations in drugs and dosage. In Minneapolis, the six-member Pharmaceutical Consultant Services was set up to offer similar services on a broader basis, counseling patients, assisting community pharmacists, and evaluating drug-usage programs for hospitals and industrial medical departments.

Daniel A. Herbert, owner of a pharmacy in Richmond, Virginia, began to supply what he called "acute pharmacy care services." Many of the people who bought their drugs from him were cancer patients who needed medicines and supplies not available in the average community pharmacy. Herbert organized his store to dispense the complex, often highly toxic, drugs that his patients needed and to monitor their complicated drug regimens, providing care that ordinarily has been available only through specially equipped hospital pharmacies. "It's a much-needed service," he said. "More and more the trend is toward outpatient chemotherapy because it saves the patient money, saves the insurance providers money and keeps the patients at home."

Another area in which pharmacists can provide specialized services is psychiatry. Many psychiatric patients have forms of schizophrenia that once required hospital care but now can often be controlled with drugs, while the patients live and work in their communities. Such treatment requires close, expert supervision—difficult to provide in thinly populated rural areas. In eight community mental-health clinics in rural Georgia, psychiatric pharmacist Wayne Copp was engaged to monitor the medication of some 200 outpatients. He kept them stabilized and out of mental hospitals. Copp's services saved the clinics some $60,000 in psychiatrists' fees alone—not to mention the much greater costs of hospitalization.

Pharmacists like Eugene White, Robert Davis, Beatrice Adreon and the others do not simply point to the future: They exemplify the elements of modern practice that identify a good pharmacist today. "Pharmacists want to use their skills," said Davis, "not just stay behind their counters." Finding and taking full advantage of a pharmacist who has that impulse is one big step in using medicines safely and effectively. ✳

The making of a professional

A generation or so ago, the local pharmacist was generally perceived as a friendly figure of authority, consulted by ailing townfolk for medical as well as pharmaceutical advice; typically, his nickname was "Doc." Today's pharmacists, by contrast, are professionals in flux—on the one hand, skilled drug experts; on the other, often underutilized because they are considered mere dispensers of pills.

Tomorrow's pharmacists are likely to be a radically new and different breed. They will be more highly skilled than ever, equipped with a body of knowledge that ranges from nuclear medicine to data banks on individual patients. But they will also be, as they were before, the community's recognized drug consultants—the persons to whom all drug queries, from patients or doctors, will be directed.

These pharmacists of tomorrow are being trained today at such institutions as the University of Maryland's School of Pharmacy in Baltimore, pictured here and on the following pages. Students at the university receive some of the most extensive training in the entire health care field. A basic bachelor's degree requires five years of study, in courses as diverse as biology and business management, chemistry and cosmetics. Classes in communication skills, given partly in a model pharmacy *(pages 124-125)*, teach students to handle probing questions from patients and physicians. And although the bachelor's degree qualifies graduates to practice pharmacy, a student can also choose from graduate programs in such specialized areas as radioactive drugs *(page 129)* and drug research *(pages 130-131)*.

Upon graduation, the newly trained pharmacist becomes a member of the new breed. According to former FDA Commissioner Jere Goyan, the pharmacist is the person doctors and consumers should "turn to for assistance and information." Said one of the new generation, a small-town pharmacist in the Eastern United States: "There's no doubt in my mind that we've got the most exciting profession going."

Using such traditional tools as mortars and pestles, fifth-year students at the University of Maryland's School of Pharmacy compound medicines in a classroom laboratory. Though most medicines are now assembled in pharmaceutical factories, pharmacists still learn how to mix drugs themselves to gain a basic knowledge of the forms and ingredients of drug preparations.

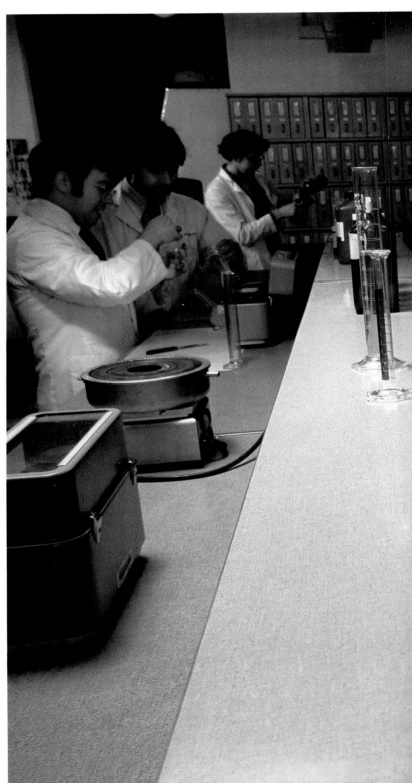

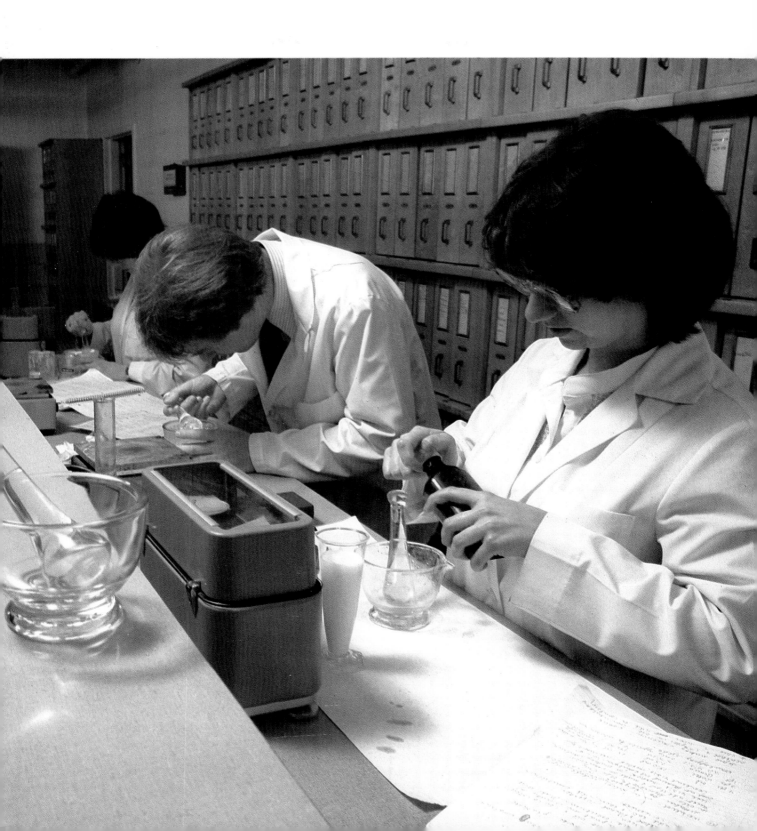

Building a broad base of knowledge

"Pharmacy has, traditionally, been conceived of as a product system," said Jack Robbins, a pharmacist who completed a survey of the profession in 1979, but the "new pharmacy has been rapidly moving away from the product system, and is becoming a knowledge system."

The trend means that today's pharmacy students master not only traditional skills but also a range of techniques unrelated to the filling of prescriptions. They learn, for example, how to take blood-pressure readings *(below),* so they can monitor a patient's drug therapy. They get direct experience in operating such devices as heating pads, thermometers, bottle sterilizers and neck braces *(right)*—enabling them to instruct patients in their use.

Much of this instruction takes place at the school's model pharmacy. There, under the supervision of an instructor, students fill prescriptions written by fictitious doctors, maintain patient drug records and counsel "patients" play-acted by their classmates. But the students also gain clinical experience in real settings, by serving internships at local hospitals. There, they work with real patients, observe doctors prescribing drugs and learn to spot adverse drug reactions and side effects.

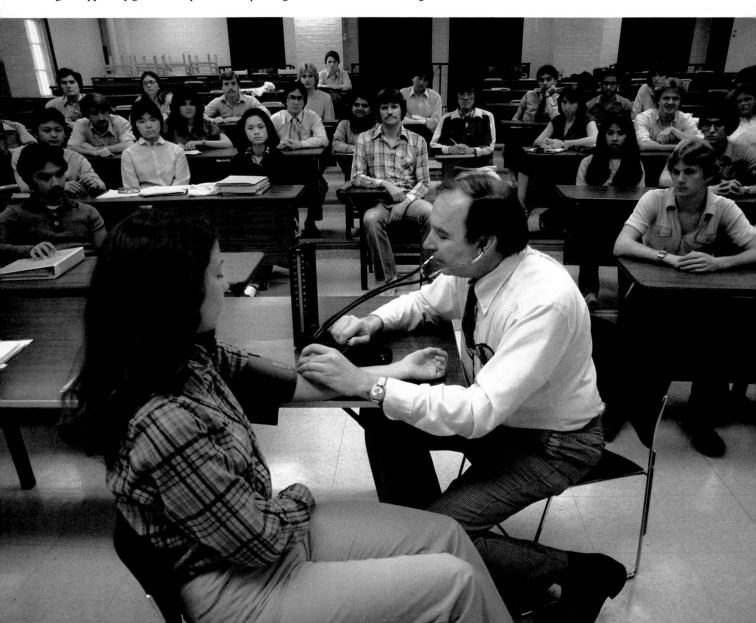

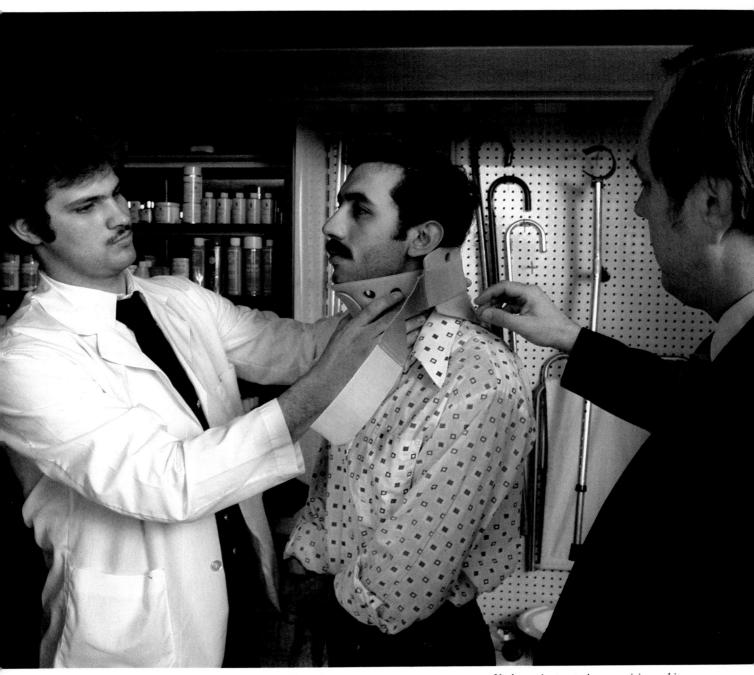

In a classroom demonstration, Professor Donald Fedder takes a blood-pressure reading from third-year student Victoria Hale. The lesson has a practical objective: In a new type of professional activity, and as a service to their communities, many pharmacists have started offering free blood pressure, urine and diabetes tests to their customers.

Under an instructor's supervision, white-coated student Mike Barnes fits a brace to a classmate's neck. Such demonstrations give students the experience they will need to operate the medical equipment most pharmacies now carry.

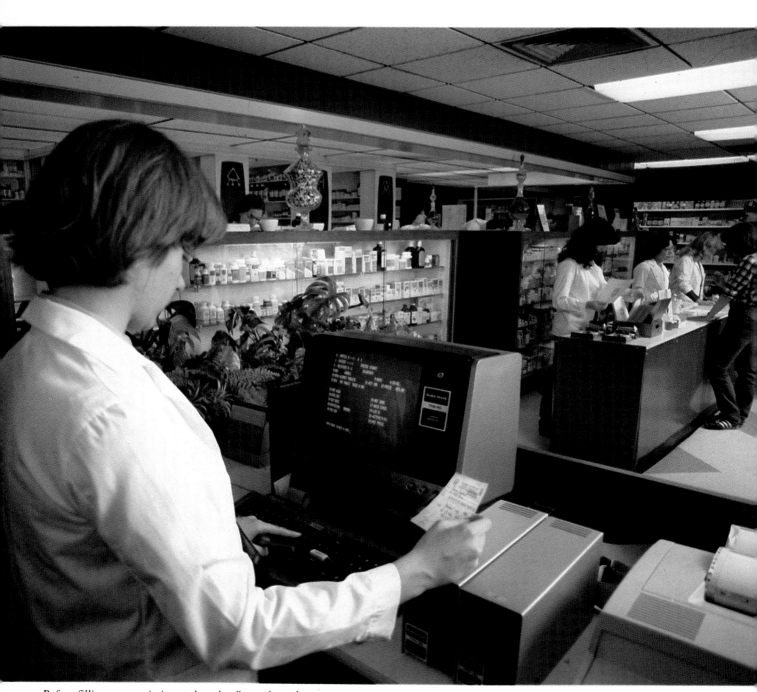

Before filling a prescription at the school's modern pharmacy, fourth-year student Anna Weikel uses a computer to check the patient's prescription record. Such data-retrieval systems make it possible for pharmacists to see at a glance a patient's normal dosage of a drug and to check the record for allergic reactions or dangerous interactions.

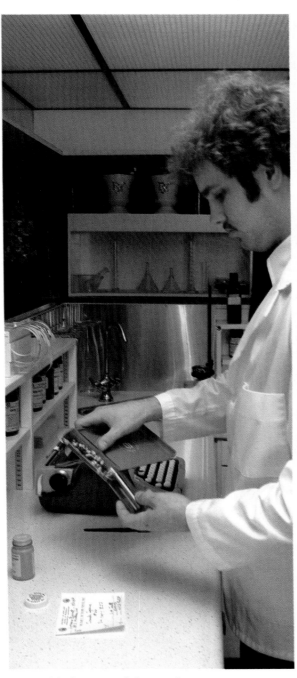

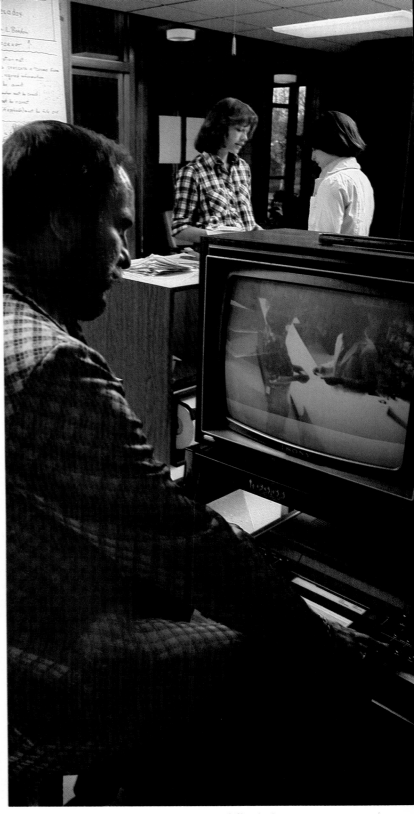

In one of the last steps of pharmacy's classic chore, Mike Barnes uses a counting tray (page 103) to fill a dispensing bottle with capsules. Surplus capsules have already been returned to the stock bottle; all that remains is to type a label.

As part of a class session on communication skills, Assistant Professor Kenneth Steiner watches a videotape recorder during the training of two students playing the roles of patient and pharmacist. After the role-playing is over, the students and their classmates will study the tape to see how well the ''pharmacist'' answered the ''patient's'' questions.

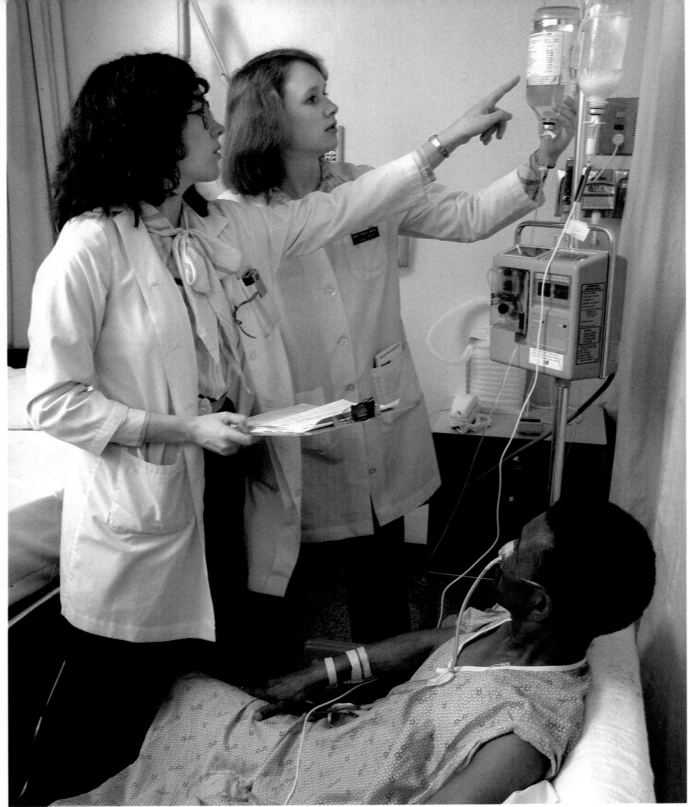

*A University of Maryland Hospital supervisor (left) shows
intern Mary-Therese Andres how to introduce nutrients and drugs
into the bloodstream through an intravenous, or IV, system.
Not only drugs, but such foods as fats (white bag) and mixtures of
sugar and vitamins (yellow bag) are often prepared by hospital
pharmacists according to a doctor's orders.*

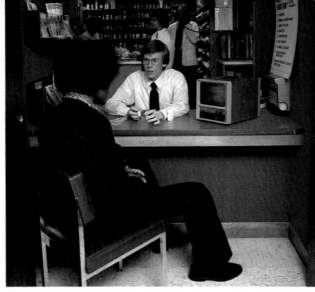

Seated behind the counter of the hospital pharmacy, student intern Alan Knudsen counsels a patient on the use of a drug. The videotape set nearby is stocked with instructional tapes on drug procedures and precautions; Knudsen can use these tapes to help him in his task.

Garbed in sterile mask, cap, gown and gloves to avoid infecting a virtually germ-free cancer-treatment room, James Hanyok, a fifth-year student, teaches a leukemia patient to give himself an injection. With the ever-increasing use of cancer drugs, many students now specialize in chemotherapy and drug counseling for cancer patients.

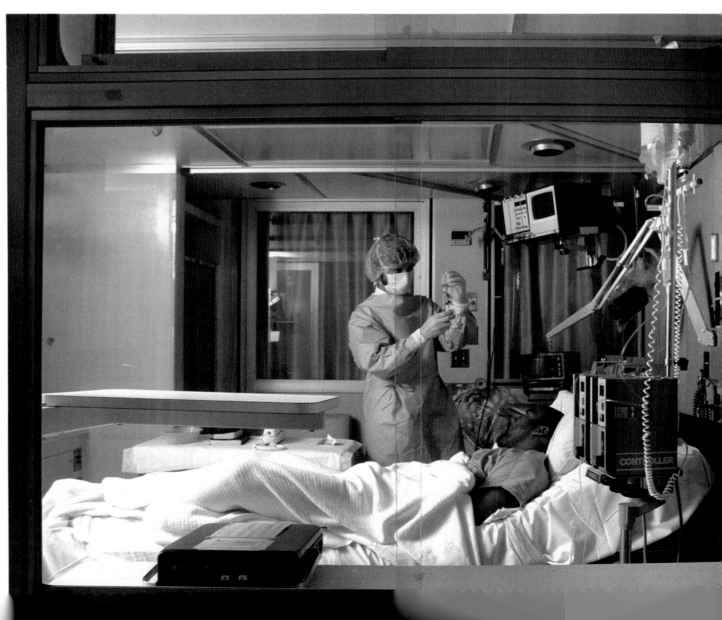

Working toward specialized goals

Though the basic skills required of the pharmacists of tomorrow can be acquired in the program leading to a bachelor's degree, many students choose to pursue the specialized on-the-job training and extra schooling offered candidates for an advanced degree. Unlike most graduate programs, the one for pharmacists is an alternative rather than an addition to undergraduate studies; a candidate for the Doctor of Pharmacy degree enters upon a course of study that takes six years to complete—a year longer than the bachelor's five. Those who graduate from the advanced program possess, among other professional skills, a greater ability

to spot and correct subtle or life-threatening responses to drugs.

For a career in research, teaching or drug development and manufacturing, rather than in pharmacy itself, the University of Maryland's School of Pharmacy also offers Master of Science and Doctor of Philosophy degrees. Students in these programs pursue their studies and research in specialized laboratories with equipment that would be found in the most sophisticated academic setting—from dose calibrators, which measure the radioactivity of cancer drugs *(right),* to gas chromatographs, which purify and isolate chemicals from tiny brain-tissue samples *(page 130).*

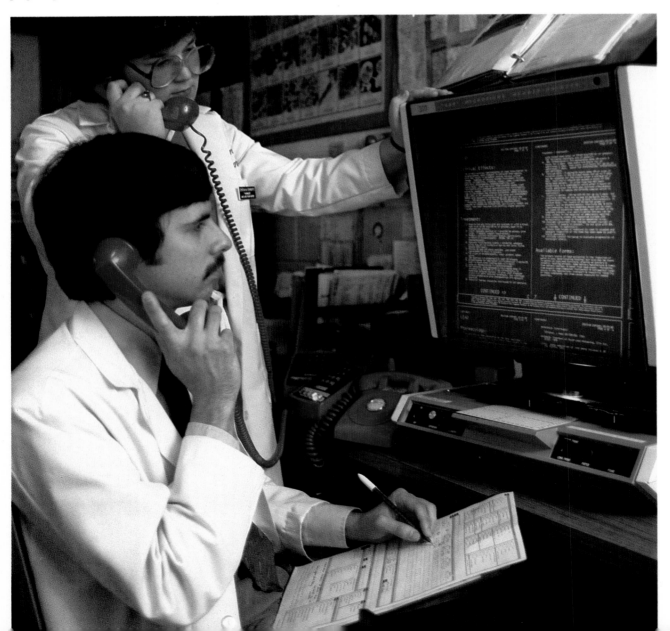

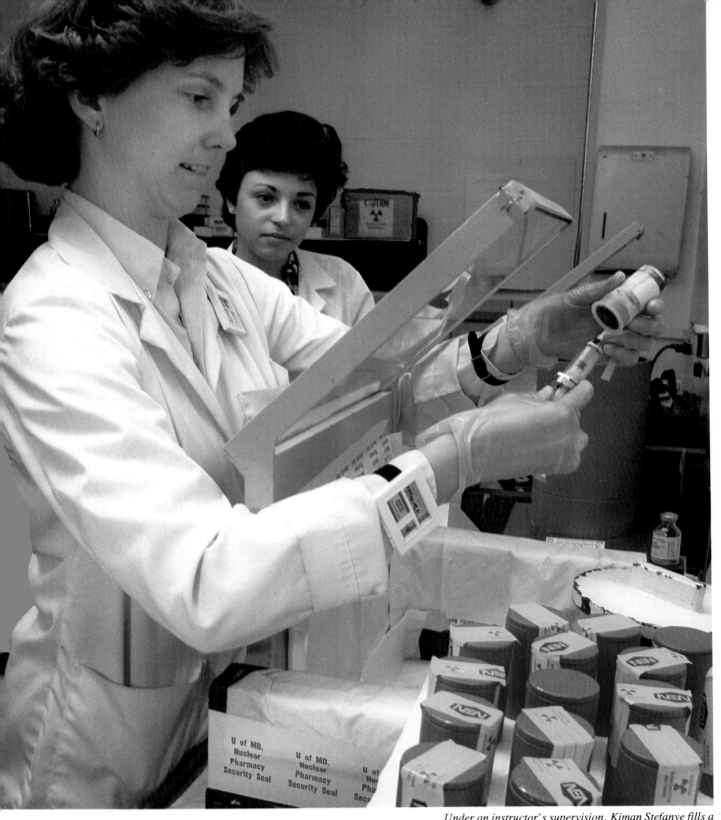

While his instructor listens in, Bruce Gordon, a candidate for the Doctor of Pharmacy degree, uses microfilmed data at the Maryland Poison Information Center to advise a caller about lead poisoning.

Under an instructor's supervision, Kiman Stefanye fills a hypodermic with osteolite, a radioactive drug used to treat bone cancer. Although the radiation levels of such nuclear drugs as osteolite are relatively low, students shield their bodies behind a leaded-glass screen and, to monitor the level of exposure, wear radiation-detection badges on their wrists and lab coats.

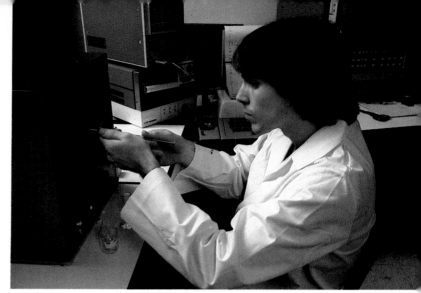

Ph.D. candidate Jerrold Adkins inserts brain tissue from a rat into a gas chromatograph. The machine will isolate a chemical thought to be involved in such diseases as epilepsy and Huntington's chorea; Adkins hopes to develop a new nerve drug by studying the chemical.

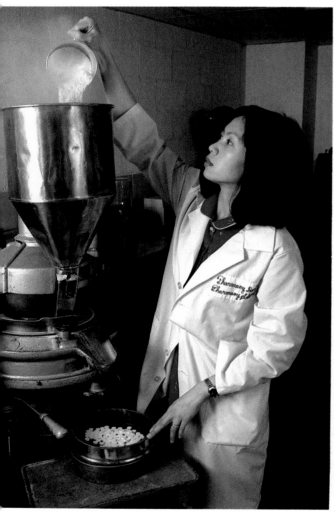

Graduate student Krongtong Mitrevej pours drug ingredients into a machine that converts the pinkish powder into tablets. The course she is taking in industrial pharmacology prepares students for careers in pharmaceutical companies.

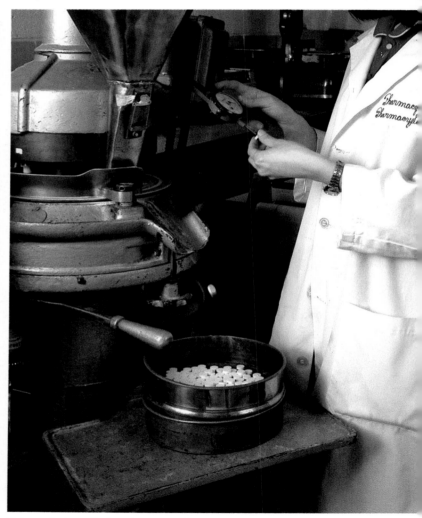

Using a device called a micrometer, the student checks the thickness of a sample tablet. Tablets must be of uniform size and density in order to ensure that the correct dosage is administered and that the drug dissolves at the intended rate.

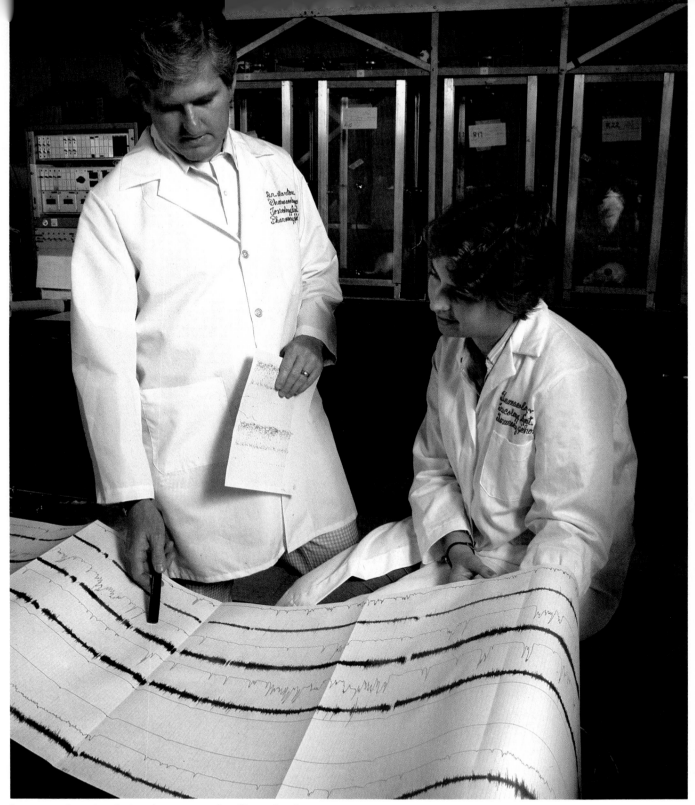

In a research project designed to compare the effects of various narcotics on the brain, Associate Professor J. Edward Moreton (left) shows pharmacology graduate student Leslie Neistadt an abnormal pattern in the brain waves of a rat. The rat's brain was permanently linked to an electroencephalograph, or EEG, by tiny electrodes implanted within its skull.

132

An internship in the real world

Only a minority of pharmacy-school graduates work for drug companies or go into research; 6 out of every 10 elect to practice in community pharmacies, where they become directly involved in patient care. The demand for care and counsel is staggering: Each year American pharmacists handle an estimated two billion drug inquiries—confirming, if confirmation is needed, the belief that pharmacists should be dispensers of drug information as well as drugs.

By choice, the pharmacist of the future will work in a pharmacy that is a professional center rather than an all-purpose store. Said one new practitioner: "When a patient meets the pharmacists in a carnival atmosphere, with TVs going and garden hoses and garbage bags all around, it takes a lot away from the image of the pharmacist." In the appropriate professional setting, even more than today, pharmacists will literally and figuratively step out from behind the compounding counter to advise patients.

"As specialists in drug therapy," said one community pharmacist, "the new pharmacist will assume comprehensive responsibility for all the drug requirements of patients. When the need arises for any drug therapy, the family physician, dentist, or other specialist will refer the patient to the drug specialist—the pharmacist—who will follow through to the termination of drug therapy." Local pharmacists of tomorrow will become the complete professionals they are trained to be—full-fledged members of the community health-care team.

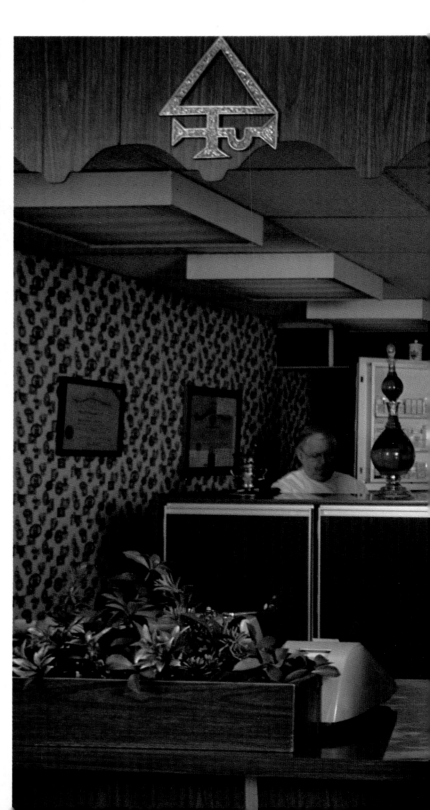

Monitored by a practicing pharmacist (rear), student intern Douglas Wright advises a patient on her prescription drug. Though this pharmacy foreshadows those of the future—it has no magazine racks, candy displays or soda fountain—decorative alchemical symbols and ruby-red show globes link it to those of the past.

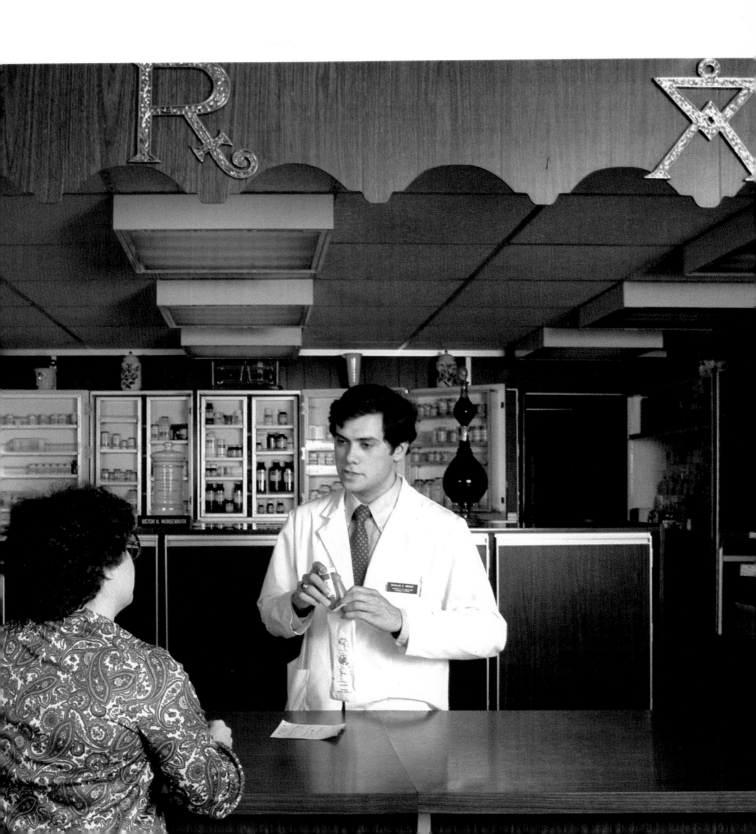

CHAPTER 6

The long, hard road from lab to pill

Playing molecular roulette to save lives
From the last move of atoms, an ulcer cure
A maze of tests to prove safety and effectiveness
Ethical dilemmas in experiments on people
Compensating for the human element
Is playing safe the cause of a drug lag?
The orphan drugs

"I just follow my nose," said Sir James Black, explaining his reputation for ingenuity in drug research. His nose led him to one of the most valuable new drugs to be discovered in the second half of the 20th Century: cimetidine — more commonly known by its trade name, Tagamet—an ulcer medicine that has changed the lives of those who suffer from stomach ailments.

The hunt for cimetidine began in September 1964, when Black and three colleagues—pharmacologist Michael E. Parsons, biochemist William A. M. Duncan and chemist Graham J. Durant—assembled outside London in the Welwyn laboratory of the noted Philadelphia-based pharmaceutical firm of Smith Kline & French (referred to informally as SK&F). Black, new to SK&F, was fresh from a triumph at another British laboratory, where he had helped develop the first of a whole family of valuable drugs called beta blockers, used to treat heart disease, high blood pressure and eye disorders, among other ailments. It was hoped that the techniques used to create beta blockers could lead to other drugs for other maladies—in particular, the common, refractory disorders, ranging from indigestion to life-threatening ulcers, that are prompted by excess stomach acid. If such a drug could be synthesized, it would help millions of sufferers all over the world.

One of the substances that cause the stomach to release acid had long been known: It is the naturally occurring compound called histamine, the same stuff that afflicts allergy sufferers with stuffy noses and itchy eyes. Underlying the research by the SK&F team was an apparent paradox: Although many of the upper respiratory reactions to histamine can be controlled or suppressed by antihistamines, those medicines are useless in retarding the secretion of stomach acid. It seemed that histamine must somehow work differently in different parts of the body—an idea that, if proved, might lead to the development of a chemical capable of blocking the acid-producing reaction to histamine by gastric cells, just as beta blockers stopped the action of catecholamines in raising blood pressure.

At that first meeting in Welwyn in 1964, expectations ran high—so high, Duncan and Parsons recalled, "we believed 'it would all be over by Christmas.' " They added: "This was to be far from the truth."

What the SK&F team hoped to be able to accomplish in a matter of months took eight years of painstaking work, involving the synthesis and testing of more than 700 different compounds; an additional four years were required before the final product could be distributed for use in Britain, and almost another year before it was approved in the United States. During those years the number of people needed to develop and prove out the drug expanded from the original four to more than a thousand specialists and many more thousands of volunteer patients; costs for the project soared to well over $65 million.

The story of cimetidine reveals a great deal about the process of drug discovery and development—a process that occasionally includes those rare, happy accidents scientists

Helping develop a new drug, a researcher checks the progress of a purification step. The murky amber solvent (bottom of tubes) holds impurities that have bonded with it; the clearer fluid retains a chemical used in a medicine for treating high blood pressure.

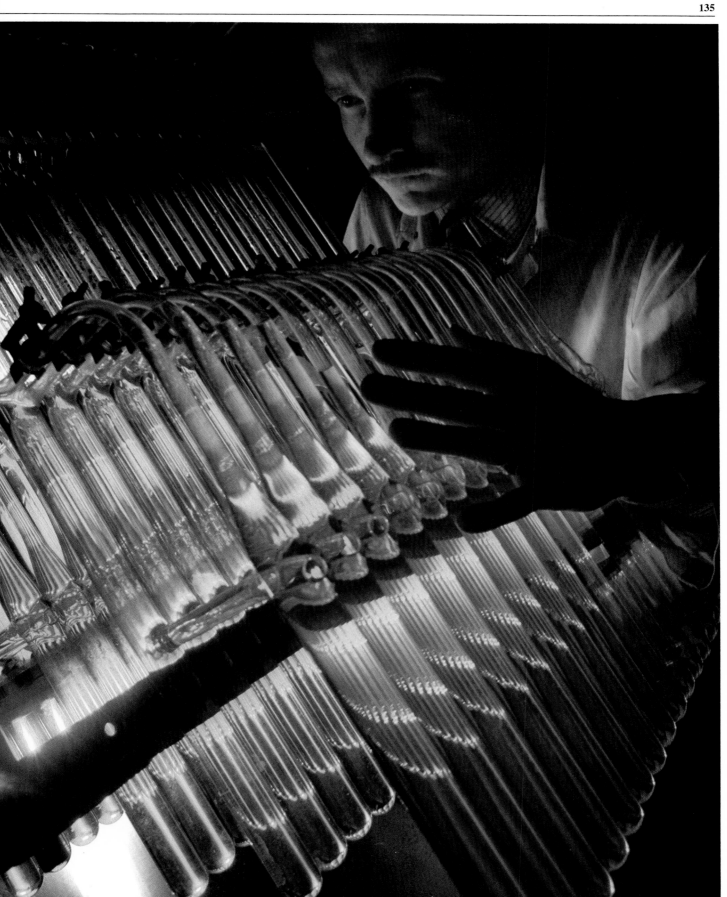

dream about, but far more often drags out into a seemingly endless ordeal of trials and errors, replete with frustrations, disappointments and slogging, repetitive work. Few compounds survive the ordeal to become part of the pharmacopeia; fewer still turn out to make a major contribution to human health.

Like cimetidine, most new drugs, including more than 90 per cent of those originating in the United States, are developed not in academic or research institutions but in the laboratories of pharmaceutical manufacturers, who have the specialized staff, the resources and the incentive required for the complex task. Finding the drug is only part—sometimes the easiest part—of the job.

The many steps from laboratory bench to drugstore shelf demand the talents not only of chemists, biologists and physicians but also of clinical pharmacologists and physiologists to study the drug's effects in living systems, veterinarians to keep test animals in good health, toxicologists to set up and carry out tests for toxicity, pathologists to examine animal organs and tissues for evidence of injury after the tests, and statisticians to compile and analyze data. Simply supplying mice, rats and rabbits for experimentation supports a thriving industry of animal breeders, who do more than $30 million in business in a typical year.

At every stage the problems facing the researchers are formidable, involving scientific uncertainty, legal restrictions, the vagaries of the human body and psyche, and often, considerations of ethical standards and religious values.

In an average year, drug-industry researchers may screen hundreds of thousands of chemical compounds for possible usefulness as medicines. Perhaps a thousand or so may prove worthy of intensive investigation; perhaps 15 of these may finally make it to market, and then often years later.

One new antibacterial drug introduced in the 1970s involved dozens of scientists working for 19 years; they screened 41,117 chemicals before they found the one they were after, sulfacytine, a drug for treating specific infections of the urinary tract. Researchers for another drug company spent two years testing more than 100,000 soil samples gathered from around the world in an attempt to come up with new antibiotics. The end result: oxytetracycline, discovered in the mold from the earth of an Indiana farm.

Most of today's medicines are not spectacular originals like oxytetracycline or cimetidine, or ''miracle drugs'' like the first penicillin or the first polio vaccines. Some are simply duplicates of older, unpatented drugs marketed under new trade names; others are new combinations of existing ingredients, or new dosage strengths or forms. Moreover, not all of the drugs that do represent significant advances are truly original compounds. Most are what pharmacologists call analogues: molecular modifications or manipulations of earlier chemicals. These analogues may be more effective than their predecessors, or safer; they may have fewer side effects, be more readily absorbed and longer-acting, or be more stable or easier for people to use.

The first penicillin, for example, has been supplemented by penicillin V, ampicillin and a host of others. Following sulfanilamide, the first sulfa drug, hundreds of variants were developed, all of them superior to the prototype.

''Drug research is a little like building a series of Tinkertoy structures in the dark, and hoping one won't fall down,'' said an industry specialist. The possible molecular arrangements and rearrangements for a given compound are virtually infinite, and a small change in the structure can make a profound difference, even determining, as with a Tinkertoy structure, whether it stands up at all.

Playing molecular roulette to save lives

To create a new compound, researchers often begin by looking at drugs that already exist in a given category; then they start trying to improve them. In developing dobutamine, a drug that increases the force of the heartbeat, scientists at Eli Lilly Company analyzed the best available heart stimulant, then set about making it better by eliminating its adverse effects; they rebuilt the molecule, step by step, eventually arriving at a compound that increased the force— but not usually the rate—of the heartbeat and did not cause either irregular heartbeat rhythms or undesirable changes in blood pressure.

Sometimes a slight molecular variation in a drug can make

it work against ailments other than the ones it was originally applied to. The tranquilizer chlorpromazine, for example, the first drug to be useful in treating seriously ill mental patients, resulted from a minor modification of phenothiazine—which had been available for decades, chiefly for use in deworming livestock.

In many cases, major new roles for drugs are revealed only after the medicines have been used for a while by humans. Certain sulfa drugs given to cure infections were found to increase the flow of urine, leading to thiazide diuretics, useful in eliminating body fluids and reducing blood pressure. Compounds used to treat Addison's disease—a hormonal disorder that causes the adrenal glands to stop functioning properly—were found to relieve the inflammation associated with arthritis; allopurinol, which was originally studied as a substance that might control the body's utilization of an anticancer drug, was found to lower levels of uric acid, the substance that causes gout.

The modification of existing compounds and the discovery of new uses for old drugs are valuable contributions to the practice of medicine, but they do not produce fundamentally new drugs. That can be achieved in only two ways. One depends on knowing what compound is needed, then building such a substance. The other is a shotgun approach sometimes referred to as random screening or molecular roulette, in which a researcher tries to invent entirely new compounds, not knowing if one will turn out to be a miracle drug, a good furniture polish or a substance that is altogether useless.

Molecular roulette turns up numbers of candidates. By testing each on animals, the experimenter attempts to find out if it has any notable effect—as sedative, stimulant, pain

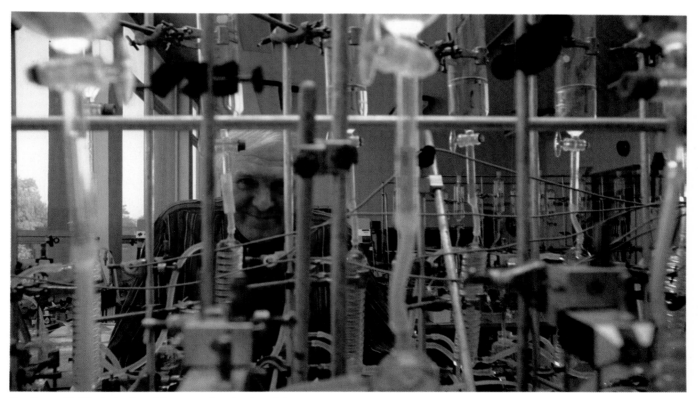

Dr. James W. Black, leader of the group that developed the ulcer medicine cimetidine, examines an experimental apparatus at the Wellcome Foundation in England, where he became director of therapeutic research in 1978. Dr. Black, led to cimetidine by his earlier creation of the beta blockers for heart disease, was knighted by Queen Elizabeth II in 1981.

reliever, or anything else. If a candidate shows some promise in these initial tests, it is subjected to more detailed screening in several species of animals to verify its effects and analyze its possibilities.

Random screening was the approach used in a major discovery by Leo Sternbach, a Polish-born chemist who had fled the Nazis in World War II and was employed at the New Jersey laboratories of the Swiss firm Hoffmann-La Roche. Sternbach was intrigued by the chemical family called benzoheptoxdiazines, which he had worked with while searching for new dyes during the 1930s. After three years of work, Sternbach came up with compound 0609, the chemical chlordiazepoxide, which when administered to mice and cats relaxed them without making them sleepy or groggy. Marketed under the trade name Librium (for ''equilibrium''), it quickly became one of the most important and widely prescribed tranquilizers.

Sternbach kept at his work; three years later, he developed another member of the family, diazepam, which proved even more effective in smaller doses and could be used for a broader range of problems. Called Valium (after the Latin *valere,* ''to be healthy''), it soon soared to the top of the list of the products most prescribed by doctors.

The other major approach to the discovery of truly new drugs, and the one that has shown the most promise in recent years, starts with an analysis of the body's chemistry, then sets out to find specific chemicals to block undesirable effects or to enhance desirable ones. Often the search begins with an attempt to make variants of a substance that occurs naturally in humans, in the hope that one of these forgeries will either hinder or help the body in its use of the natural chemical. Because this direct approach aims at a specific problem, it is theoretically more likely to succeed.

Plotting a triumph over stomach acid

It was this sort of head-on scientific attack that led ultimately to cimetidine. Sir James Black and his fellow scientists based their strategy, already proved effective in the development of the beta blockers, on the concept of agonists and antagonists *(page 80)*. They knew that histamine triggers the release of acid in the stomach because it is an agonist, a substance whose molecular shape interlocks with receptors on the surface of a body cell to stimulate a specific reaction. They were looking then for an antagonist, a chemical imposter whose characteristics were close enough to those of the agonist to allow it to fit partially into the same receptor, producing no response itself but blocking the agonist from occupying the site.

The scientists were familiar with the molecular structure of the histamine agonist as well as the structures of various antihistamines. Moreover, they knew that a single agonist can sometimes react with two different kinds of receptors, requiring not one, but two compounds to successfully block it from both sites. Finally, they knew that it is possible to alter the chemistry of an agonist in order to transform it into its own antagonist.

The scientists took as their starting point the basic structure of the histamine molecule, atoms arranged in a pentagonal ring. They then stripped away the groups of atoms hung on this ring and replaced them with other groups, in this way reshaping histamine into something slightly different. One of these offspring, they hoped, might work in blocking the action of its parent. To determine if each new compound had any effect on biological activity, either as an agonist or an antagonist, each was tested on pieces of live tissue taken from laboratory animals.

This work eventually produced evidence that there were indeed two different histamine receptors: one responsible for stuffy noses, the other for secreting stomach acid. This proof came from tests of two histamine variants, which differed only in a minor molecular detail. Both were agonists, but they stimulated different histamine reactions. The receptors affected by the first were designated H_1, the acid-stimulating receptors affected by the other were termed H_2. Sir James's idea seemed confirmed. ''It was our first 'Eureka' day,'' a company research official recalled.

Two more years passed before identification of the first antagonist that was even slightly effective on the H_2 receptors—and it turned out to be a compound synthesized at the very start of the research. Its action had gone unrecognized until, belatedly, one of the project's key tests—for acid in rat stomachs—was improved.

By the end of 1968, the researchers had synthesized a still more promising chemical, SK&F 91486. Tinkering with the molecular structure had enhanced its activity as an antagonist—enough to convince the scientists that they were on the track of something big.

But the parent company in Philadelphia, meanwhile, was growing impatient. The team had expended almost five years during which it "sank a lot of dry holes," recalled Robert Dee, the company's chairman. "We were within an ace of calling it quits. We then decided to go one more year." Faced with this deadline, team-member William Duncan, by then research director at Welwyn, decided to concentrate all of the laboratory's resources on the histamine project, letting others lapse.

By mid-1970, barely within the deadline set by the home office, and after the British team had passed the 700 mark in compounds synthesized and tested, they came up with SK&F 91923, burimamide. It proved to be the best H_2 antagonist yet. Although its potency was still too low to make it a useful drug, the scientists decided to go ahead with tests on healthy human volunteers—a step they could take on their own in Britain but not in the United States, where governmental approval is required.

A notice was placed on the bulletin board at Welwyn; the first to volunteer were Duncan himself and Dr. Robin Ganellin, another member of the expanding research team. Under careful monitoring, histamine was injected into their veins to stimulate an increase of gastric acid; this was followed by administrations of burimamide. As expected, the new chemical caused a slight reduction in the acid level in the volunteers' stomachs.

Seventy more compounds later, the research team arrived at a viable successor, SK&F 92058, metiamide. It was hardly different from burimamide—tacked onto one corner of the histamine ring was a methyl group (a carbon atom surrounded by three hydrogen atoms), and tucked into a long chain at another corner was an extra sulfur atom. This minor reshuffling, though, increased potency tenfold. "Things really began to swarm," recalled Bryce Douglas, the company's chief of research and development.

By now the team had mushroomed to 150 or more persons, constituting most of the staff at Welwyn. In April 1973, Britain's Committee on Safety of Medicines issued a certificate permitting clinical trials in actual ulcer patients.

With the trials of metiamide, an effective and apparently safe blocker of stomach acid, James Black considered his goal achieved. He left the team at Welwyn to follow his nose to other challenges.

From the last move of atoms, an ulcer cure

But there was a problem with metiamide. As widespread trials in ulcer patients got under way, a few reports of a condition known as agranulocytosis began trickling in. Agranulocytosis is caused by a drop in the infection-fighting white blood cells and is marked by lesions of the throat and other mucous membranes. While the numbers of subjects affected were small and the condition cleared up when metiamide was withdrawn, the isolated cases were alarming enough to give the company pause. After consultations in Philadelphia, Douglas telephoned Duncan at Welwyn: "Cease clinical work on metiamide. Where is your successor compound that won't give us this problem?" Sadly, the researchers put the new drug back on the shelf. The trial certificate of metiamide was revoked by the British authorities—except for emergency use in ulcer patients whose lives were endangered.

"These were indeed dark days, and concern for the future was now greater than it had been at any time since the program started," Duncan recalled. But development had already begun on a promising backup, SK&F 92334, cimetidine. It differed from metiamide only in the replacement of one sulfur atom by a group of carbon and nitrogen atoms. Cimetidine, happily, proved safer and twice as potent as metiamide in laboratory tests, and a new clinical trial certificate was obtained.

Then one day in late 1975, a call was received at the Welwyn labs from a doctor who had heard of the new chemical and who had a seriously ill ulcer patient he was treating with metiamide. The patient's white-blood-cell count had plummeted because of the drug, discouraging further use. But to save his life, his secretion of gastric acid somehow had to be suppressed. Was it possible to get an emergency supply of cimetidine?

It was not an easy decision. This would be no carefully controlled clinical test, but a high-risk experiment on a man who was desperately ill. What if cimetidine did not work? What if the patient died?

Duncan consulted the SK&F review board in Philadelphia, which had to approve all tests in human subjects. After weighing the evidence accumulated about the drug, the review board decided to make what one of its members characterized as "a leap of faith." A supply of cimetidine was rushed to the hospital in England, where it was substituted for metiamide. The patient's white-blood-cell count rebounded, and within a few weeks his ulcer had healed. Although a single case could not count for much, the inventors of cimetidine were elated.

From this point, development of the new drug gathered momentum. As more and more trials on groups of patients confirmed both the efficacy and safety of cimetidine, British health authorities issued the company a product license in 1976. Further trials were arranged in France, West Germany and other countries.

Marketing of the new drug began under the trade name Tagamet, devised by combining the second syllables of the words "antagonist" and "cimetidine"; it was decided to manufacture the tablets in a pale green color—which was deemed psychologically soothing to patients—and to stamp them with the code number T-13.

If cimetidine had achieved acceptance with relative ease in Europe, however, far sterner tests lay ahead in the United States. The standards of the U.S. Food and Drug Administration (FDA) for acceptance of new drugs are among the most exacting in the world. Their rigor stems in part from the thalidomide disaster of the early 1960s (page 20)—the United States narrowly escaped the thousands of birth deformities caused by the drug in other nations. On the heels of the thalidomide furor, an aroused Congress passed stringent new laws, demanding that "substantial evidence" of the safety and efficacy of any new drug be presented before it can be approved for sale.

A maze of tests to prove safety and effectiveness

To enforce these laws, the FDA requires that tests be carried out prior to approval of a new drug for general use. Because of their stringency and extent, the tests are costly and time-consuming—but they provide significant safeguards and are increasingly being adopted by other countries.

Three different kinds of tests are stipulated by the FDA. First are animal toxicity tests to find out how poisonous the drug is—all drugs can be harmful in some way because to be effective they must interfere with normal body processes. Clinical trials on gradually increasing numbers of patients follow toxicity tests to prove efficacy. Finally, long-term studies attempt to uncover subtle effects that may not appear until after protracted use.

Animal tests are often challenged by those who claim that differences in body structures and biological processes limit their value. But the fact is that such tests are not only necessary to avoid endangering human lives, but also revealing.

The fundamental similarities between humans and other animals, particularly other mammals, are more striking than the surface differences. And fast-breeding creatures such as mice, rabbits and rats can be genetically selected to yield strains of identical animals with specific characteristics. One strain of mice, bred to be unusually vulnerable to high levels of blood sugar, gives a quick check of drugs meant to treat diabetes.

Furthermore, it is possible to choose animals to match a particular drug, selecting those species that are most likely to respond to that type of drug the way humans would (pages 141-143). In the testing of cimetidine, rats and dogs—whose bodies absorb, metabolize and excrete substances in much the same way that human bodies do—were extensively used.

Had sufficient testing of animals been required prior to the reforms of the 1960s, many authorities argue, some serious miscalculations might have been avoided. Chloroquine, for example, an antimalarial drug developed during World

Of mice and men: how drugs are tested

Since about the turn of the century, a Noah's ark of animals—from skittish rats *(right)* to docile sheep *(page 143)*–have been used by scientists to develop new, safe medicines for humans. Some tests on animals have represented dramatic medical turning points: In the 1950s, for example, scientists inoculated rhesus monkeys with an experimental polio vaccine, then injected them with polio virus; they found that the vaccine worked and was safe. Other experiments, though less spectacular, have been considered no less crucial. Indeed, all drugs now must be tested on animals before they can be released for human use.

The animals most commonly used for drug research are rodents and rabbits. They are prolific breeders, and their breeding can be laboratory-controlled. This ensures that all generations of animals are genetically similar and, thus, that drugs will affect them similarly. More important, these small mammals often react to drugs as humans do.

To test some drugs and vaccines, however, larger animals are better. In tests of drugs for the viruses that infect the nervous system and brain, cats and dogs are used because they contract viral nerve infections like those of humans. Yet the most prized—and costly—test animals are primates, such as chimpanzees and monkeys, for they resemble humans in anatomy and physiology more closely than any other creature, great or small.

An electrode implanted in its brain, a laboratory rat awaits a pleasurable electrical stimulus—to be delivered each time it presses a lever. Once the rat learns the task, it will be given a test drug to see if the compound alters its reactions.

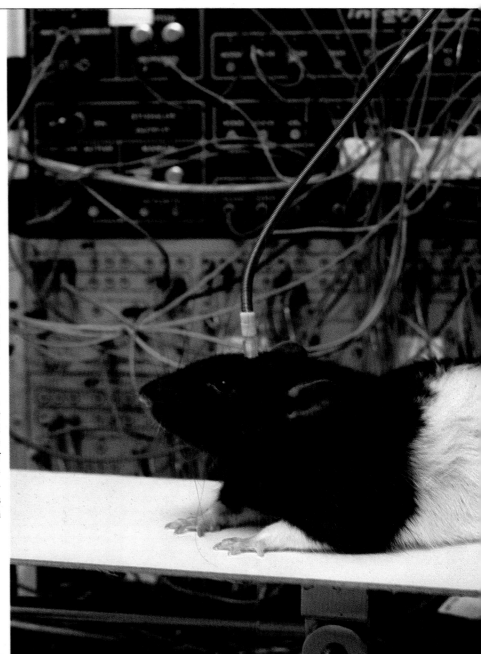

A scientist studies the movements of a lobster being used for tests of a drug that paralyzes animal parasites such as roundworms. The lobster's nerve fibers resemble those of parasitic worms, but they are larger and easier to study.

A cat learns to feed itself by pressing a lever that releases food into a tray beneath the floor of its cage. Later, the cat will be injected with an experimental antihistamine and watched to see if it presses the lever fewer times than before—an indication of a suppressed appetite. Cats, like humans, are among the few species whose appetites slacken after doses of most antihistamines.

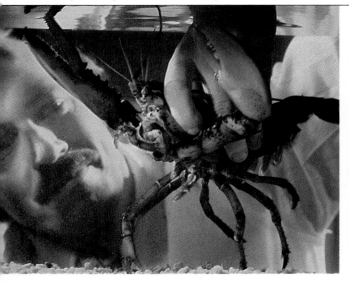

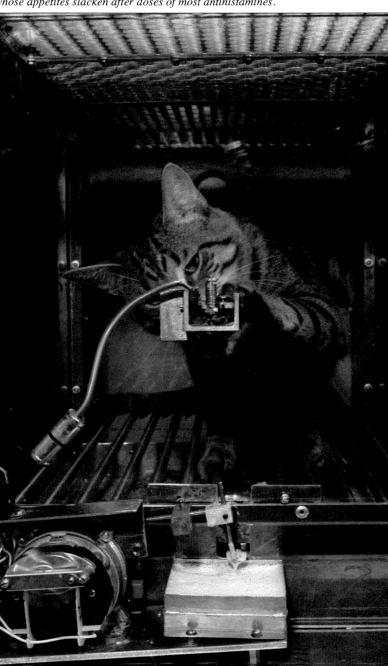

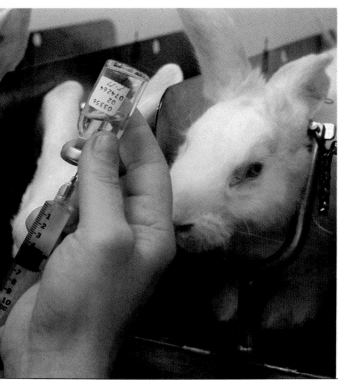

Their heads gently harnessed, rabbits in stainless-steel stalls are about to receive injections of an antibiotic that is being tested to see if it produces fever. Rabbits were chosen because they are very sensitive to fever-causing chemicals.

Using a tongue depressor, a scientist examines the teeth of a
rhesus monkey, a seemingly unwilling subject, in the course of an
experiment to test the effects of certain drugs on tooth decay.
The teeth of the rhesus and other monkeys and apes are similar to
those of humans, a fact that qualifies these animals as ideal
subjects for dental research of this kind.

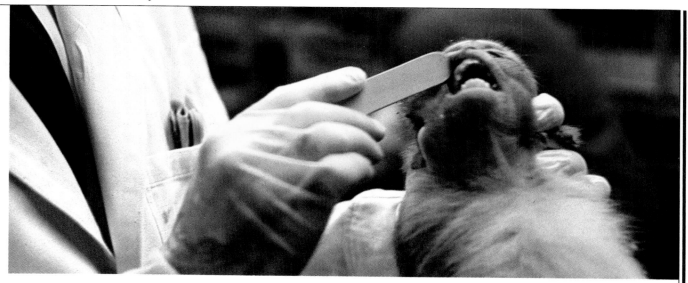

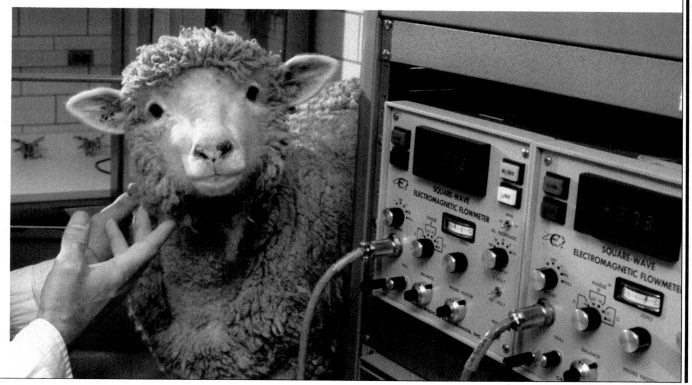

After receiving an experimental drug that lowers blood
pressure, a sheep calmly permits a research scientist to take a
pulse reading from its neck, which has been partially shorn of
wool to make the arteries easier to find. The drug was being tested
for its effect on the sheep's kidneys and urinary system, which
are similar to those of human beings.

War II, was tested only in relatively small dosages, and was declared safe. Later, when larger doses were found to be useful in treating arthritis and were prescribed without additional testing, it was learned that chloroquine in larger amounts is toxic to humans.

Learning about such hazards is the first aim of drug trials, and it obviously requires animals. These studies are divided into acute (short-term) and chronic (long-term) experiments. In the former, increasingly large doses of the drug being tested are given to different groups of animals, and researchers watch for adverse affects. They want to determine how much of a compound must be given the animals—usually several species are used—to kill them.

By averaging the results of such trials, it is possible to calculate how big a dose is required to kill 50 per cent of the animals receiving that amount of a drug; this is known as the "lethal dose fifty," or LD50. To provide a rough gauge of relative safety, the LD50 is divided by the median effective dose, or ED50, the amount needed to accomplish the drug's desired effect in 50 per cent of the same species of animals. These calculations yield what is known as the drug's margin of safety. The closer the ratio is to 1, the more dangerous the compound.

If the ratio is deemed satisfactory for the type of drug in question—a high risk might be acceptable in the case of a new cancer drug, but unacceptable for, say, a new cold preparation—the experimental compound is then submitted to "subacute" tests. In these, pathologists search for evidence of drug-induced changes in livers, kidneys, and other organs and tissues obtained from animals.

Animals are also essential for long-term chronic studies because they mature rapidly enough for the actions of a drug to be followed during a lifetime. This is important for compounds that will have to be taken steadily over long periods for chronic diseases.

The possibility that a drug might cause cancer or, if taken by pregnant women, harm an unborn baby is carefully examined. Sedatives, painkillers and stimulants are tested to determine how addictive they may be. Said FDA pharmacologist, Dr. Vera C. Glocklin: "The whole philosophy behind animal testing of drugs goes back to the canary-in-the-mine concept—using animals to determine what is safe for humans."

Vital as testing in animals continues to be, however, opposition and criticism persist. Antivivisectionists consider it unnecessary, cruel and immoral. Others join them in questioning the morality of sacrificing animal lives, even to save human lives. "If we acknowledge that animals have independent value," said Thomas Regan of the Department of Philosophy and Religion at North Carolina State University, "can we justify using them for research? Biological differences don't mark moral boundaries." Some scientists have similar doubts.

Animal testing cannot of course predict all human responses to a drug. Compounds that affect emotions and the mind are understandably difficult to evaluate because methods have not been perfected to detect mood changes in animals. Although no reasonable substitute for animal testing has yet been found, no one argues that it is perfect or that it can be a final step. "Man is unique," emphasized science-policy analyst William Lowrance. "No animal is the best model for man." In the end, the only fully reliable test for drugs intended for human beings must be one conducted with human beings.

Ethical dilemmas in experiments on people

At first glance, testing drugs on people seems absurdly simple: Choose someone subject to a disease, give him a compound that promises to make the disease go away, then see what happens. This process, in fact, was followed for centuries. Its potential for error and tragedy came to light only during the dramatic expansion of research that followed World War II. Human beings, it turned out, make poor subjects for experimentation. They may vary inordinately one from another in the reactions of their bodies and their minds; both kinds of variation can have a remarkable impact on the results of experiments. And ethical values can assume overriding importance.

The dimensions of these difficulties were made clear by Dr. Henry K. Beecher, who was for 30 years director of the anesthesia laboratory at Massachusetts General Hospital. In

Rat fetuses, stained to highlight skeletal structures, are examined for abnormalities caused by a drug that was administered to the parent animal. Such tests help weed out new drugs that could be unsafe for pregnant women and their unborn babies.

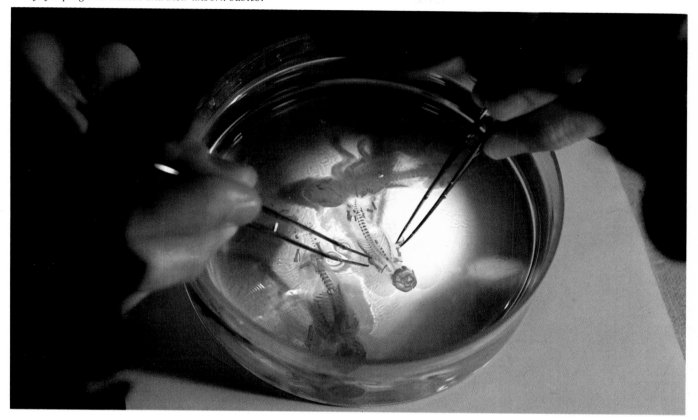

an article for the New England Journal of Medicine in 1966, Dr. Beecher cited case after case that raised disturbing questions about the then-current practices in human testing. He wrote: "Evidence is at hand that many of the patients in the examples to follow never had the risk satisfactorily explained to them, and it seems obvious that further hundreds have not known that they were the subjects of an experiment although grave consequences have been suffered as a direct result of experiments described here."

In his examples, Dr. Beecher carefully avoided giving any names; his goal was to call attention to questionable practices, not to indict individual researchers. Among the experiments he cited: In Brooklyn, live cancer cells were injected into 22 patients who, according to a review of the experi-

ment, were informed only that they would be receiving "some cells." During another experiment, involving persons with streptococcal respiratory infections, 109 patients were denied penicillin treatment (although it was established that such treatment by injection could prevent them from developing a serious aftereffect, rheumatic fever). Instead, they were given dummy pills so their responses could be compared with those of patients receiving penicillin.

Perhaps even more disturbing than Dr. Beecher's examples were later revelations about a long-term U.S. Public Health Service study conducted in Tuskegee, Alabama: A number of black men who suffered from syphilis were given little treatment for 40 years so that researchers could trace the progress of their disease.

These questionable practices and many others like them came to light at a time of mounting concern about the moral, ethical and legal problems inherent in the use of humans for medical research. Actually, the concern was as old as the practice of medicine itself. Nazi experiments on unconsenting prisoners, especially Jews in the death camps, had shown that such concerns were not just theoretical.

The first principle of the Nuremburg Code, developed during the war-crimes trials of Nazi doctors, states that "the voluntary consent of the human subject is absolutely essential." Moreover, the code prohibits experiments where "there is an *a priori* reason to believe that death or disabling injury will occur" and warns that the risks should never exceed "the humanitarian importance of the problem to be solved by the experiment."

Despite postwar attempts to translate those principles into practice, Dr. Beecher and others found numerous examples of doubtful ethics in the conduct of experiments with humans, including research involving prisoners, mentally retarded children and fetuses. At the heart of the issue was the concept of "informed consent."

Reformers argued that research on human subjects should not be allowed to proceed unless the patient is made fully aware of the nature of the experiment, as well as its risks and dangers, and has explicitly agreed to participate. Coercion of any kind should be forbidden, they insisted.

Largely as a result of public concern for the rights of experimental subjects, informed consent is now an absolute requirement. Those involved in an experiment must know the risks before it begins. The sponsors of any new drug are required to guarantee that impartial, broadly based committees—including not only physicians, but lay members such as lawyers and clergymen—will closely review the proposed research to ensure that the rights and safety of human volunteers are fully protected.

Such requirements, necessary as they are, may complicate human testing. Subjects for trials may be more difficult to recruit: Experimentation on mentally retarded individuals and prisoners, if not forbidden, is now at least discouraged because those people are considered more susceptible to coercion than members of the general population. Their exclusion adds to the complexity of assembling the large numbers of human subjects required before trials of a new drug are completed.

These trials are divided into three phases. Phase I seeks to establish the safe dosage range and to observe how the human body reacts to and excretes the drug. In order to minimize danger, the tests in this phase are performed on a relatively small number of subjects—between 20 and 80 healthy volunteers. Phase II tests the drug's effectiveness in treating the condition for which it is intended and requires a larger number of volunteers, in most cases between 100 and 300. Phase III is designed to simulate how a compound will be employed in general medical practice and can involve thousands of human subjects. For example, 15,000 persons were used in Phase III of the tests for the first oral contraceptive, 20,000 for the first oral antidiabetic drugs, and more than 3,000 for cimetidine.

Phase I testing is safe—no cases of permanent harm attributable to a test drug during this first stage are known to the FDA. Serving as a screen, Phase I eliminates some of the newly synthesized compounds. Cimetidine made it through with little difficulty, but a study cited by the Pharmaceutical Manufacturers Association showed that, on average, only one out of eight drug candidates that are subjected to human testing actually reach the public. The remainder are abandoned because they either fail to produce the desired effects or cause undesirable side effects.

Compensating for the human element

The drugs that pass Phase I, usually restricted to healthy volunteers, must then prove they can help hospital patients and outpatients who suffer from the conditions the medicines are designed to treat. The fact that an experimental drug appears to make the patient well is not sufficient. The researchers must take into account the remarkable ability of the human body to heal itself. The body's internal repair mechanisms, unaided, usually can take care of numerous illnesses, sometimes even ulcers. To allow for self-healing, most drug trials include a control group—subjects who get either no medicines at all or substances different from the one under test.

Controls permit comparison, so that one treatment can be judged against another, but such comparisons can prove misleading unless carefully managed. First, the separate groups must be matched so that the characteristics of the controls resemble those of the subjects actually receiving the test compound. Obviously it makes little sense to compare youthful controls with elderly test subjects. One of the cimetidine tests was rejected by the regulatory authorities because characteristics of the two groups of patients who took part in it were not sufficiently comparable to provide meaningful results. Even genetic differences may influence the effects of drugs.

Attention to such detail in the conduct of trials seems elementary, but how far this care must be carried may be hard to determine. During the development of the malaria drug primaquine, for example, researchers noted its untoward effect on some blacks—those who have a deficiency of an enzyme that prevents primaquine from attacking red blood cells might suffer from severe anemia. But not until primaquine had been in widespread use for several years was the same effect discovered in some Caucasians of Mediterranean ancestry, and in some Asians as well.

Human beings, no matter how carefully selected and matched, are too variable to permit simple comparisons between test and control groups. Chance enters into the results. If 60 per cent of the test subjects receiving a drug got well while just 50 per cent of those in the control group got well in the same period of time, the 10 per cent difference could be due to chance.

Researchers need objective criteria to decide whether the difference is meaningful: The solution is to analyze the results statistically, using the mathematical tools originally developed for gambling games, later applied to the testing of such things as electric light bulbs and artillery shells, and now used for public opinion polls.

Such calculations indicate whether a test result is "statistically significant" by figuring the odds against its having arisen by chance. If the odds against chance are 20 to 1 or greater, most experts accept the results as statistically significant. Significance depends mathematically on the number of subjects in the test and in control groups and on the magnitude of the difference in results.

Statistical analysis cannot make up for one of the peskiest sources of error in drug testing: the influence of the human mind. Some studies are of the "open" type, in which the drug is simply tested on willing patients who know exactly what they are taking. Open studies—which were relied on almost exclusively until the 1950s—are still the rule with new cancer drugs, substances that are generally so toxic they cannot ethically be administered to anyone unless he is told what he is getting; such a drug is given only to cancer victims who have failed to respond to other therapies and to whom it offers some hope. Open trials are also necessary for drugs being tried on dangerous illnesses such as severe infections or heart irregularities; in these cases, the patient must be informed that an experimental substitute is being used for the standard treatment.

Open testing is avoided whenever possible because it can yield equivocal and sometimes confusing results. The mind can affect the body's reactions to internal and external stimuli, altering responses to drugs. One expression of this problem of mind over matter is the placebo effect: the potential of human beings to turn a dummy pill into an actual cure.

During the testing of cimetidine, the placebo effect was in full evidence. In one trial of over 650 ulcer sufferers, 40 per cent of those given placebos were cured in four to six weeks.

To reduce the placebo effect, researchers must attempt to keep subjects in both test and control groups ignorant of the nature of their treatments. Such secrecy is difficult to maintain. Inquisitive volunteers who have used a similar drug before may sense differences in the appearance, odor or taste of the medicines they are given. Subjects may also respond to unconscious hints from doctors and nurses concerning their role in the experiment. Even side effects such as headaches, nausea and constipation may occur more frequently in one group than another—this has been especially true, for some reason, among those in placebo groups.

The most common technique for canceling the placebo

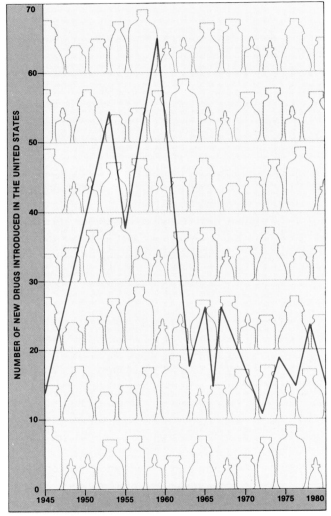

When U.S. requirements for testing drugs were stiffened after 1960, the number of new prescription remedies put on the market —which had increased sharply over more than a decade— suddenly dropped (above). Stricter regulation saved Americans from several medicines that had been approved abroad but later were proved dangerous, and it discouraged the introduction of imitative drugs. But the elaborate tests also delayed some valuable drugs until long after they were common elsewhere —the effective remedy for heart disease, propranolol, could not be prescribed until 1976, 11 years after its first use in Europe.

effect is the so-called controlled, double-blind study, in which an experimental compound is tested against a placebo administered in a form identical in appearance and taste to the drug. Patients, doctors and nurses are kept in the dark, or "blind"; neither doctors or nurses know which patients are getting which kind of pill. The test drug and the placebo are identified by code numbers known only to the pharmacists who have made up the preparations.

Difficulties in matching individuals in the two groups are sometimes circumvented by means of the "crossover" technique, in which Group A gets the real drug for a week while Group B receives the placebo. Then the procedure is reversed. Crossovers, however, can be used only for conditions, such as high blood pressure or diabetes, that remain relatively stable for a period of weeks so that the effects of the real drug and the placebo can be reliably compared; such tests are useless for infections that develop and change rapidly.

FDA regulations require that most drugs be subjected to at least two controlled experiments of the double-blind type, carried out by physicians thoroughly familiar with the disease in question and specially trained for this kind of research. The actual number of studies required for a given drug will depend on the urgency of the need for it as well as on how clearly the first few studies demonstrate its superiority over a placebo or control substance; the greater the difference in the healing rate between the two, generally speaking, the fewer the number of subsequent studies that will be needed before testing proceeds to the final phase.

In the case of cimetidine, 16 major double-blind trials were performed in the United States and Europe, but nine were rejected as either incomplete or flawed. In addition, SK&F submitted the results of open studies by European physicians. Although there were some tests in which the gap between cimetidine and the placebo was fairly narrow, in other trials the findings tilted heavily in cimetidine's favor; sometimes a healing rate of 80 to 90 per cent was recorded for the drug compared to 25 or 30 per cent for the placebo.

Interestingly, the narrower margins of effectiveness for cimetidine were recorded in the United States, where ulcer sufferers commonly consume more antacids (with their acid-neutralizing effects) than do their counterparts abroad—and were allowed to continue doing so during the trials. In all the tests, moreover, the incidence of adverse reaction to cimetidine was remarkably low, mainly involving mild diarrhea in 1 per cent of those receiving the drug, and muscular pain, dizziness or rash in an even smaller percentage—findings that have been borne out in continued testing on thousands of patients.

One unexpected and amusing bit of evidence also came to light in the course of the cimetidine trials: Doctors reported that some of the patients taking the drug had begun putting on unaccustomed weight. It developed that these long-suffering people felt so well—for the first time in years—that they were happily consuming second helpings of their meals. After reviewing the mounting evidence, Dr. Roger Crossley, SK&F's director of clinical research, announced to a meeting of his colleagues: "Gentlemen, we now have a new side effect: gluttony!"

If Phase II trials indicate that a drug is likely to be useful in treating a disease—and if continued testing in animals turns up no evidence suggesting a potential for long-term harm—human testing then enters Phase III. The objectives: to prove efficacy beyond a reasonable doubt, but mainly to identify any infrequent but possibly serious effects that have not yet come to light.

To accomplish this, the drug is tested under much the same conditions that would exist if it were approved for general use. It is given to a larger number of patients in hospitals and outpatient clinics; it is administered by their regular physicians. Generally, several cases of a particular adverse reaction must be observed before the reaction can be linked to the test compound.

Some adverse reactions are so uncommon that to test for them would require inordinate numbers of patients and years of study; to conclude that a drug produced undesirable effects in 1 of 100,000 patients, for example, researchers would have to give it to roughly a million persons in all—which would be virtually the same as approving it for general marketing. Larger-than-normal Phase III studies have been deemed necessary in some special cases involving unfamiliar

drugs with a potential for widespread and repeated use; even so, the greatest numbers of humans tested have been 15,000 for the first oral contraceptive and 20,000 for the initial oral antidiabetic drug.

Phase III testing may take as long as two years or more. If a drug survives the trial, the pharmaceutical company sponsoring it then proceeds to the final step: It submits a New Drug Application (NDA), requesting legal permission to market the product. This NDA is accompanied by exhaustive documentation that must include everything known about the medicine as well as complete records of animal and human studies. The paper work involved in preparing this documentation can be mountainous.

A few months before cimetidine's NDA was submitted in October 1976, another drug company submitted an arthritis-medicine application that amounted to 125,000 pages bound into 307 volumes; included were the detailed results of almost six years of testing in humans. Cimetidine's own documentation comprised enough volumes of data to fill a pickup truck.

Is playing safe the cause of a drug lag?

The amount of time and effort that must be expended before a new drug may be licensed in the United States can be frustrating to drug-company researchers and executives. According to a study carried out by the General Accounting Office, it took an average of 20 months to win approval for "important" new drugs and 36 months for other drugs. Overall, an average of 23 months was required to obtain approval for a new compound in the United States, the report found, compared to some 12 months in Switzerland and only five months in the United Kingdom.

But caution has proved valuable. From the mid-1960s to the mid-1970s, for example, the FDA was criticized for its failure to permit the marketing of beta-blocking heart drugs, the development of which played such a key role in the creation of cimetidine. The FDA's suspicions were later proved at least partially correct. One chemical in the beta-blocking group was ultimately found to be "markedly carcinogenic," and the manufacturer withdrew its application.

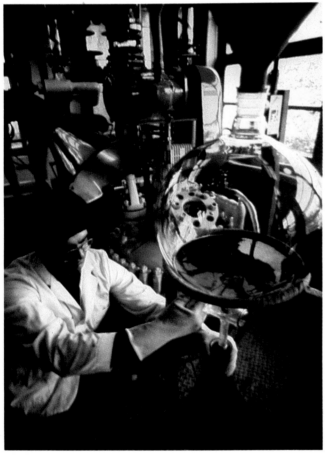

At a Pfizer, Incorporated, research plant in Connecticut, a chemist used a device called a separatory funnel to isolate the active ingredient of an experimental drug. A mixture containing the ingredient is agitated in the bulbous section, then allowed to settle; lighter, unwanted components rise to the top and a concentrated drug solution is drained out at the bottom.

A second beta blocker, which was marketed in Europe while the FDA considered its application in the United States, caused what an FDA official described in an interview as "the biggest catastrophe since thalidomide." Among the effects noted in some patients who took the drug: blindness, severe skin disorders and an intestinal blockage known as peritoneal fibrosis, requiring difficult surgery to correct. Later, other beta blockers, tested and found to be safe, were approved by the FDA.

Such conservatism, valuable as it may be, exacts a price. The years of testing and bureaucratic delays add substantially to the cost of bringing a new drug to market, thus driving up the prices consumers must pay. Moreover, the critics point out that during the 1970s, nine out of ten drugs for which New Drug Applications were filed won eventual approval, notwithstanding the strict review procedures. While this could well be the result of the FDA's insistence on thorough testing, prompting drug companies to screen out less promising candidates early, the drug industry and many physicians insist that more testing does not necessarily provide more safety.

The most serious charge against the regulatory process is that it has prevented or unduly delayed the introduction in the United States of therapeutically valuable new drugs widely available elswhere. In 1971, Dr. William Wardell, a New Zealand-born, Oxford-trained physician practicing in the United States, was astonished one day during hospital rounds to discover that his American colleagues had never heard of an asthma drug, metaproterenol sulfate, that had been used in England since 1963. Disturbed by this apparent "drug lag," as he called it, Dr. Wardell began to document its extent; he later reported to a Congressional committee that in the 17 years following passage of the post-thalidomide reforms in the United States, almost four times as many new drugs had become available in the United Kingdom as in the United States.

Such comparisons often ignore the new drugs' value to health. "By that standard," FDA Commissioner Donald Kennedy told a Congressional committee in 1979, "the difference between nations is relatively small. For example, during the period 1975 through 1977, England approved approximately 26 new therapeutically significant entities while the United States approved 37.''

The orphan drugs

But useful drugs are delayed not only by the high costs of exhaustive testing—carried out with no guarantee the drug will be approved—but also by limits on demand or profitability. These so-called orphan drugs treat relatively rare diseases and may also be drugs that are natural substances rather than laboratory creations; these natural compounds cannot be patented by a single company to prevent competitors from cashing in on its research.

Typical of the orphan drugs is the white powder called L-5-hydroxytroptophan (L-5-HTP), a natural substance that is extracted from a bean and cannot be patented. It helps curb myoclonus, a rare neurological disorder that leaves its victims bedridden, unable to speak or control their muscles.

One sufferer of myoclonus is Sharon Dobkin, a concert pianist who obtains L-5-HTP from a chemical-supply house. In this raw form, the drug's strength and purity are unreliable, so her physician, a myoclonus specialist, compounds and encapsulates the drug himself. Because his work is considered experimental, he must submit lengthy reports to the FDA; because no drug firm will support his research, he must apply each year for government or foundation grants. The nerve-racking frustration was summed up by Sharon Dobkin: ''It is extremely difficult to live from month to month, never knowing if the medication you depend on to keep your life style normal will be available.''

Victims of ailments as rare as myoclonus are not the only ones who have suffered while orphan drugs awaited legal adoption. A more common disorder is epilepsy, which affects some two million Americans. In the 1960s it was discovered that valproic acid was successful in the treatment of epilepsy. Valproic acid proved an effective anticonvulsant and for many users caused less severe side effects than other commonly prescribed drugs. But not until 1978, almost 10 years after it won official approval in France, was it available in America.

Cimetidine was no orphan. Ulcers are so common that the sales potential for a drug that could treat them effectively was great. And cimetidine was a unique, patented compound. Its credentials included carefully controlled studies on well over 3,000 patients in 26 countries, an outpouring of enthusiastic reports from physicians who had prescribed the drug in Phase III testing, thousands of scientific papers published in professional journals, and several major symposia attended by ulcer specialists from around the world, during which the new compound was favorably discussed. Under a rating system adopted by the FDA in 1974 to speed approval of drugs promising important therapeutic gains, cimetidine was given an ''A'' priority, the highest, and put on a ''fast track'' through the bureaucracy.

Final approval still did not come within six months (the statutory deadline the FDA was supposed to meet for top-priority drugs). But on August 17, 1977—10½ months after the application was submitted, and 13 years after James Black assembled the original team in their laboratory outside London to find out why ordinary antihistamines do not inhibit the production of excess stomach acid—cimetidine was cleared for release in the United States. Two years later its domestic sales alone totalled $250 million.

If anything, the medical and economic success of cimetidine intensified the search for best-seller drugs at the expense of the less glamorous, less lucrative medicines. Yet the story of this drug demonstrates that, despite all obstacles, the combination of an idea and tenacity—and money—can still improve life for millions of people.

Modern techniques of drug research, combined with conservative requirements for proof of safety and effectiveness, may work slowly, but they work to the general benefit. Said one physician: ''The sooner we look at medicines realistically for what they are—remarkable healing tools with plenty of risks and limitations as well as benefits—the better off we will be. And the sooner all of us in the system—drug makers, pharmacists, doctors, patients, politicians, consumer activists—stop regarding each other as born adversaries, the sooner we will be able to work more effectively toward the goal of better health.''

Medicinal treasures of the deep

There is nothing terribly unusual about scuba divers exploring the spectacular undersea sights of the Caribbean, of Australia's Great Barrier Reef or of the waters off the coasts of Florida, Hawaii and Southern California. But what now draws some divers into these and other deeps is most unusual—a search for ocean plants and animals that might yield valuable drugs.

The search already has borne fruit. One chemical—tetrodotoxin, obtained in Japanese coastal waters from puffer, porcupine fish and sunfish—was found to have 160,000 times the painkilling power of cocaine; this nonaddictive drug is now used as a painkiller for some victims of cancer and leprosy. Another drug, cytosine arabinoside, was modeled after a substance found in a type of sponge; it now helps treat leukemia.

Less than 1 per cent of today's commercially available drugs come from the sea—but few of the oceans' 500,000 or more species have been tested for pharmacologic activity. The pace of that testing is quickening. "Drug companies finally are realizing that there are some good new compounds" in the sea, said Professor William O. McClure, former director of the University of Southern California's marine-drug research center. To get at them, marine biologists, chemists, pharmacologists and microbiologists take to the world's waters, descending to depths as great as 200 feet and collecting plants and animals by hand. Once gathered, the specimens customarily are transported to laboratories ashore, where they are tested for their ability to alter processes of life, the fundamental criterion for a drug.

One such exploration, conducted by University of Oklahoma researchers Pushkar Kaul and Francis Schmitz, led to the discovery of dactylene, a chemical obtained from the bottom-dwelling mollusks called sea hares. Dactylene may inhibit the breakdown of barbiturates in the human body, enabling doctors to prescribe smaller and safer, yet equally effective, doses of these sedative drugs. Another substance—monoalide, extracted from a Pacific sponge by researchers from the University of California—may be useful against arthritis.

One of the most exciting leads so far has come from the otherwise unexceptional sea squirt. Extracts from the sea squirt have demonstrated some potential to combat cancer and a remarkable ability to overcome the ubiquitous herpes virus, which causes skin eruptions and is implicated in many far more serious conditions. These extracts, pointed out researcher Kenneth L. Rinehart of the University of Illinois, "are among the most active antiviral compounds yet found."

Searching for marine life that might yield chemicals for drugs, a diver (top), silhouetted against the deep blue of the Caribbean, nears a large barrel sponge. "We look for any organism that grows stuck to the bottom in a plantlike mode," said marine-drug researcher William O. McClure. Such stationary organisms probably have survived because they possess chemical defenses, some of which might have medicinal properties.

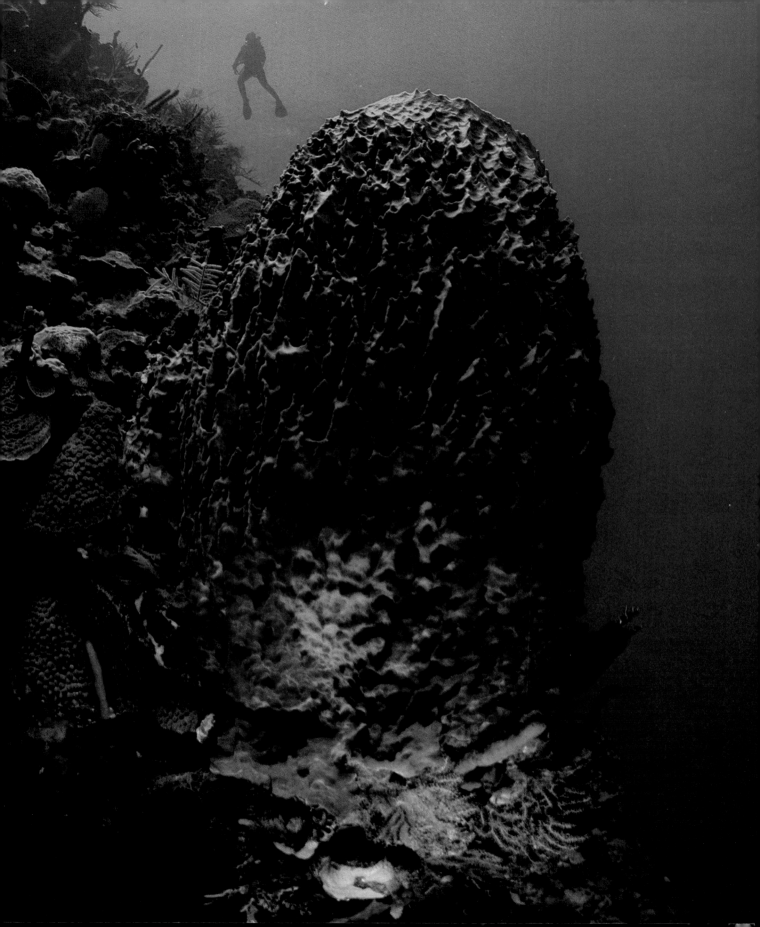

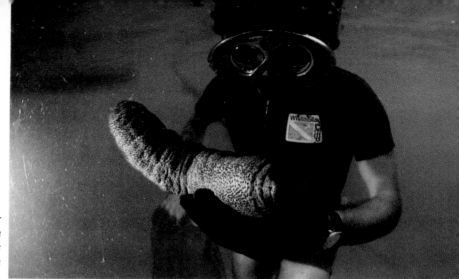

His hand gloved for protection, a diver prepares to surface with a sea cucumber, an animal that protects itself from predators by releasing holothurins—poisons that in tests proved toxic to cancer cells.

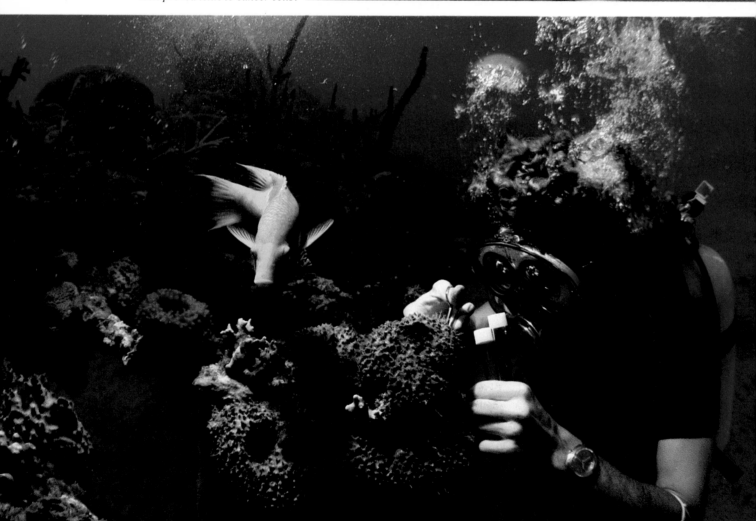

As a handsome Spanish hogfish whips past, a diver in the Caribbean snips off part of a soft sponge that he will place in a vial for later testing. Chemicals from a Caribbean sponge yielded the cancer drug cytosine arabinoside; now those from many other sponges are being examined for their effects on tumors and on the cardiovascular and central nervous systems of mammals.

A diver grabs a bouquet of sea whips from the ocean floor. Some of these soft corals contain biological regulators, or hormones, called prostaglandins; in humans, prostaglandins help control blood pressure, muscle tension and ovulation. Drugs containing marine prostaglandins have been tested as contraceptives and as remedies for peptic ulcers and asthma.

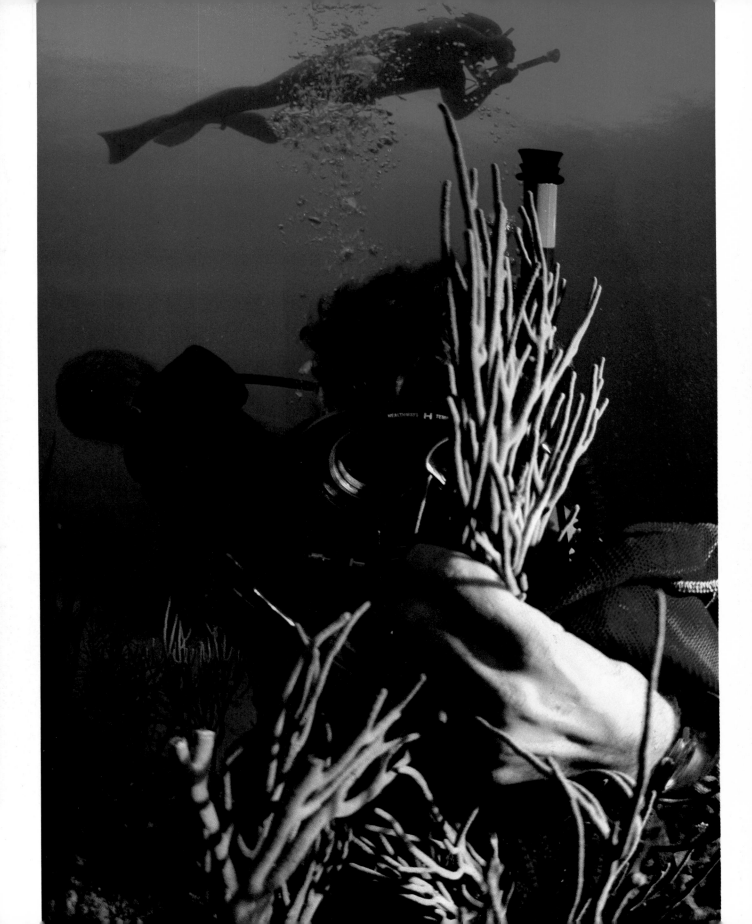

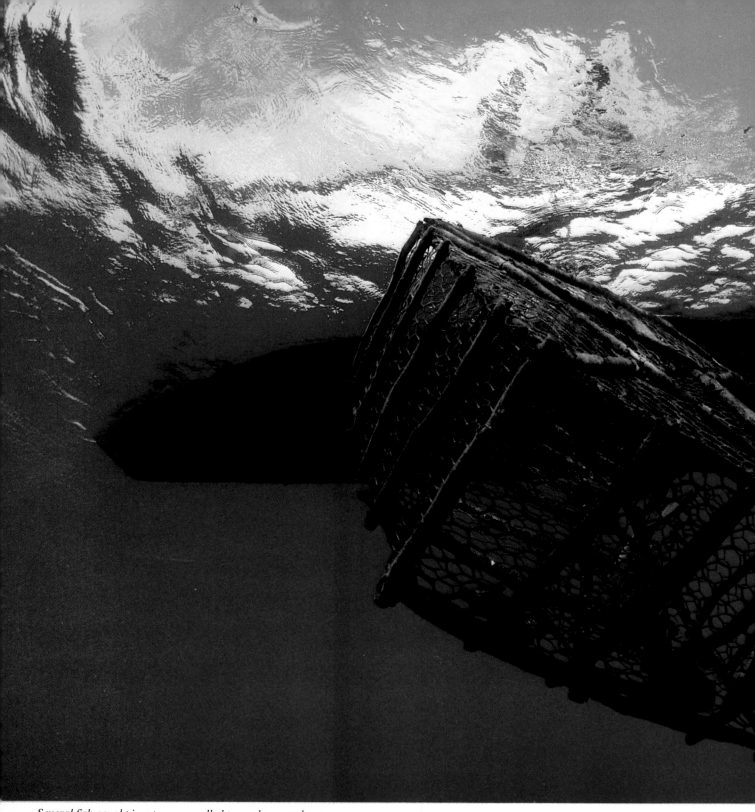

Several fish caught in a trap are pulled toward a motorboat that will take them to a shore laboratory. Fish are not considered as useful a source of drugs as marine plants and stationary animals: Most fish are not as easy to collect in large numbers, nor are they as likely to possess chemical defenses.

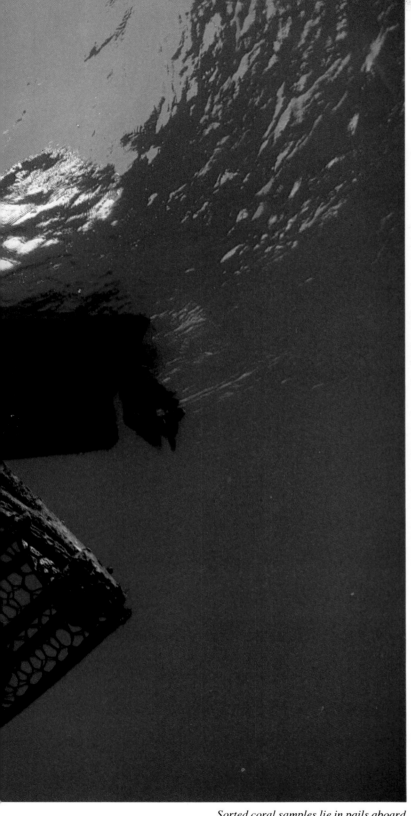

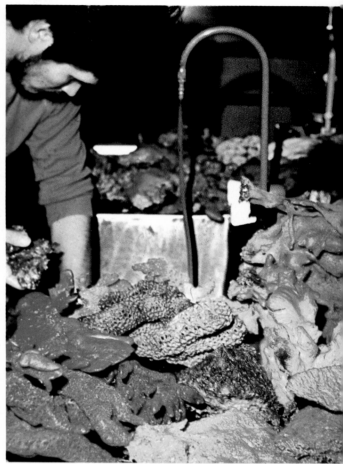

A biologist sorts sponges in an Australian laboratory. Among the tests these specimens underwent were experiments to see if they held chemicals that would kill bacteria.

Sorted coral samples lie in pails aboard the White Lightning III, an American research boat. The specimens—some preserved in alcohol—will be carried ashore and tested for drug potential.

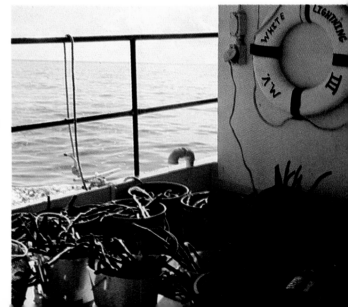

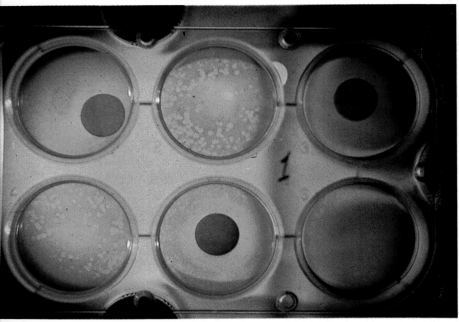

A tray with cultures of animal cells combined with herpes virus shows the varying effectiveness of six marine chemicals. At top middle, bottom left and bottom right, the virus (white speckles) won out. At top left and right the chemicals (red discs) killed both the cells and the virus. The most promising chemical, at bottom middle, killed most of the virus, but left a bright corona of unharmed cells.

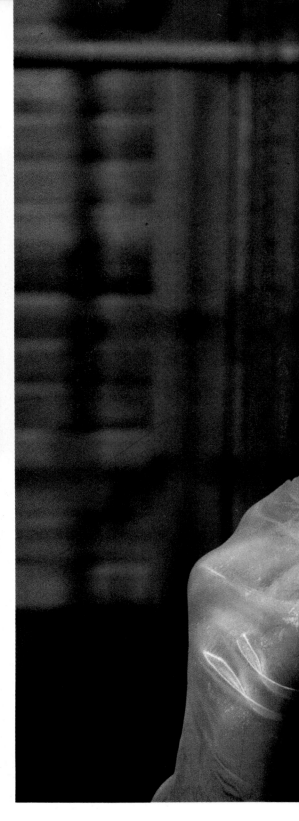

Wearing sterile gloves, a scientist studies a culture dish containing a vertical strip of a microorganism from the intestinal fluid of a surgeonfish. The microorganism was tested against three different bacteria strains (horizontal strips) for antibiotic effect. In this test it worked against the bacteria in the two lower strips, inhibiting their growth near the chemical.

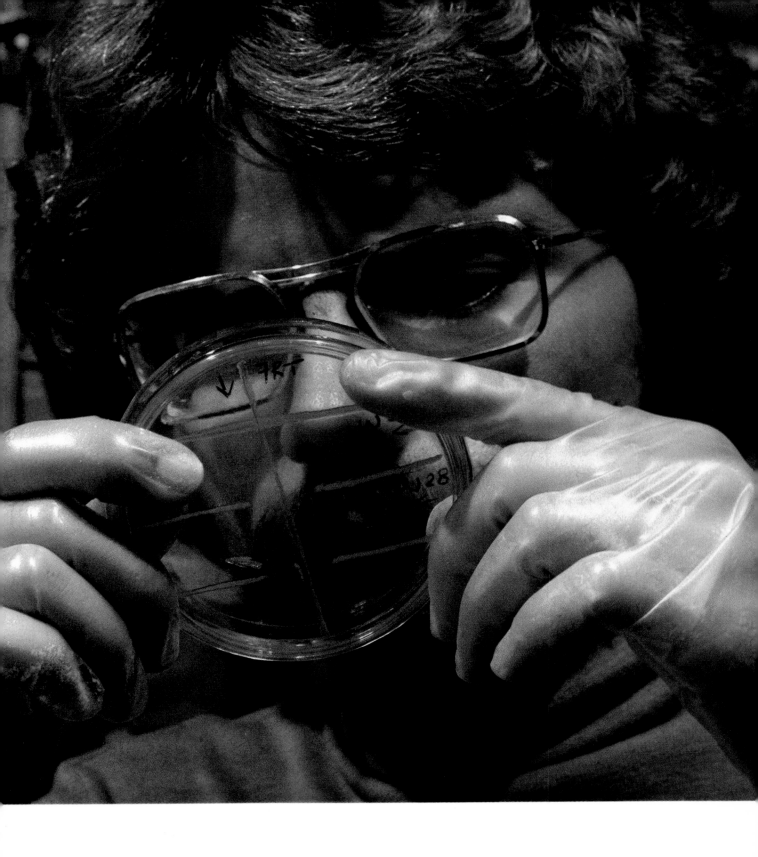

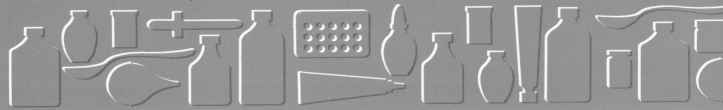

The modern drugs of choice

Of all the accomplishments of medical science, none may rival in positive impact those in the field of pharmacology. Drug researchers have provided doctors with thousands of compounds to prevent, cure or control ills that were, in earlier times, either chronically annoying, debilitating or fatal.

Listed and described in the table that begins below are 102 of today's most frequently employed medicines, prescription and nonprescription. The table, prepared by Christopher S. Conner, Director of the Rocky Mountain Drug Consultation Center, is a representative sampling of the most commonly used drugs.

The drugs are listed by the generic chemical names of their active ingredients, with a few of the most common brand names beneath. Preparations that contain more than one compound are designated by an asterisk. Drugs that require a doctor's prescription are noted by the familiar pharmaceutical insignia, Rx.

To use the table, look up the generic name of each of a drug's active ingredients, which can be discovered either by checking the drug's label or by asking your pharmacist. The table's second column describes the intended effects of the drug; the third and fourth columns list the minor and major side effects that a user might encounter. Because drugs affect individuals differently, some users may experience many side effects while others suffer few or none. If you do notice any unanticipated, persistent or severe side effects, call your doctor.

The table's fifth column provides special information—tips on how to avoid side effects, and warnings of dangers that might not be side effects as such, but that might arise through the drug's action or your reactions to it. To see whether the drug you plan to take interacts with others—and many do—consult the special companion table that appears on pages 88-89.

DRUG	Intended effect	Minor side effects	Serious side effects	Special cautions
ACETAMINOPHEN **DATRIL** **TYLENOL**	Relieves headaches and neuralgia; relieves pain in muscles and joints; lowers fever	Dizziness; diarrhea and upset stomach	Liver damage or hepatitis; reduced white-blood-cell and platelet counts	Consult doctor before taking if you have liver disease. Inform doctor of sore throat, fever, bleeding or bruising—signs of reduced blood-cell counts.
ALLOPURINOL (Rx) **ZYLOPRIM**	Reduces uric-acid levels	Diarrhea; nausea; drowsiness; stomach pain	Skin rash; kidney stones; tingling in hands and feet; liver damage; reduced platelet and white-blood-cell counts.	Consult doctor before taking if you have kidney disease. Drink plenty of fluids after taking this drug. Inform doctor of sore throat, fever, bruising or bleeding—signs of reduced blood-cell counts.
ALUMINUM **HYDROXIDE** **DI-GEL*** **GELUSIL***	Neutralizes stomach acid	Constipation; flatulence; nausea; vomiting	Severe constipation; fecal impaction	Consult doctor before taking if you have kidney disease. Take within one hour after meals to maximize duration of effects.
AMINOPHYLLINE (Rx) **AMINODUR*** **SOMOPHYLLIN***	Eases breathing in asthma, bronchitis and emphysema	Nausea; vomiting; nervousness; diarrhea; headache	Irregular heartbeat; confusion; persistent vomiting; muscle tremors; convulsions	Consult doctor before taking if you have heart disease or a peptic ulcer. Inform doctor if you experience tremors or if you vomit up blood or material that resembles coffee grounds.
AMITRIPTYLINE (Rx) **ELAVIL** **ENDEP**	Relieves depression	Drowsiness; dry mouth; dizziness; tiredness; headache	Blurred vision; chronic and severe constipation; difficulty urinating; irregular heartbeat; reduced white-blood-cell counts; fainting; liver damage; seizures	Consult doctor before taking if you have asthma, heart disease, epilepsy, glaucoma, liver disease, or if you are recovering from a heart attack. Use caution while driving or operating heavy machinery. Inform doctor of sore throat or fever—signs of reduced white-blood-cell counts. This drug may take several weeks to work. Do not discontinue abruptly after prolonged use.

* Combination drug. Refer also to other active ingredients on label.

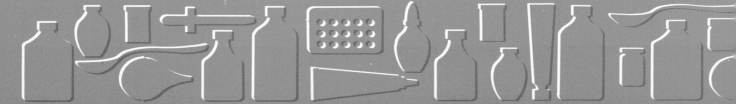

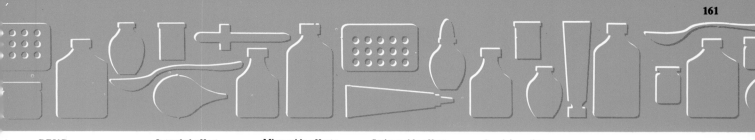

DRUG	Intended effect	Minor side effects	Serious side effects	Special cautions
AMOXAPINE (Rx) **ASENDIN**	Action similar to AMITRIPTYLINE			
AMOXICILLIN (Rx) **AMOXIL**	Cures bacterial infection	Nausea; diarrhea; vomiting	Allergic reactions, such as skin rash, itching, wheezing; inflammation of the colon (colitis)	Consult doctor before taking if you have any allergies, particularly to any type of penicillin, or if you have kidney disease.
AMPICILLIN (Rx) **AMCILL** **POLYCILLIN** **PRINCIPEN**	Action similar to AMOXICILLIN			
ASPIRIN **MANY BRAND** **NAMES**	Relieves headaches and neuralgia; relieves mild to moderate pain in muscles and joints; lowers fever; reduces inflammation; prevents blood clots that cause heart attack and stroke	Upset stomach; ringing in the ears; mild drowsiness	Bleeding and erosion of the stomach lining; development or activation of gastric ulcer with prolonged use; liver and kidney damage; slowed blood clotting; allergic reactions	Consult doctor before taking if you have hay fever or asthma—you may experience an allergic reaction marked by nasal congestion, wheezing or shock. Stop taking one week before surgery unless otherwise directed. Consult doctor before taking if you have bleeding disorders, are taking drugs to prevent blood clots, have an ulcer or are pregnant. Do not take tablets that smell like vinegar—the odor indicates the presence of acetic acid, a by-product of aspirin decomposition that can irritate the mouth and stomach. Minimize stomach irritation by taking with a glass of milk or water.
CALCIUM **CARBONATE** **TITRALAC** **TUMS**	Action similar to ALUMINUM HYDROXIDE			
CARBAMAZEPINE (Rx) **TEGRETOL**	Relieves neuralgia: controls epileptic seizures	Drowsiness; dizziness; nausea; vomiting; dry mouth; blurred vision	Reduced platelet and white-blood-cell counts; severe skin rashes; liver and kidney damage; confusion	Consult doctor before taking if you have liver or kidney disease or if you are pregnant. Inform doctor of sore throat, bruising or bleeding—signs of reduced blood-cell counts. Use caution while driving or operating heavy machinery.
CEFACLOR (Rx) **CECLOR**	Cures bacterial infections, particularly of the ear in children	Diarrhea; nausea; vomiting	Allergic reactions, such as skin rash, hives, itching, wheezing	Consult doctor before taking if you have any allergies, particularly to any form of penicillin. Take with food if stomach upset occurs.
CEFADROXIL (Rx) **DURICEF**	Cures bacterial infections, particularly of the urinary tract	Diarrhea; nausea; vomiting	Allergic reactions, such as skin rash, hives, itching, wheezing	Consult doctor before taking if you have any allergies, particularly to any form of penicillin. Take with food if stomach upset occurs.
CEPHALEXIN (Rx) **KEFLEX**	Action similar to CEFADROXIL			
CHLORAMPHENICOL (Rx) **CHLOROMYCETIN** **MYCHEL**	Cures bacterial infection	Nausea; vomiting; diarrhea	Reduced platelet and red- and white-blood-cell counts; eye pain or loss of vision; numbness or weakness of hands or feet; confusion	Take as directed until drug is gone, even if you feel better in a few days. Inform doctor of sore throat, fever, bleeding, bruising or tiredness—signs of reduced blood-cell counts. Inform doctor of eye pain, or of tingling or weakness in hands or feet.

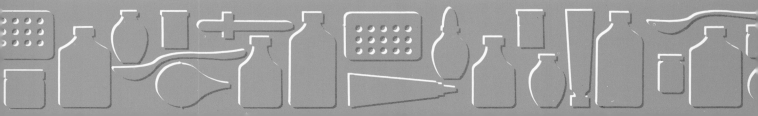

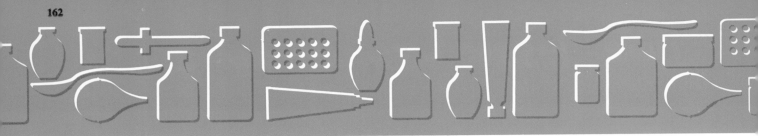

DRUG	Intended effect	Minor side effects	Serious side effects	Special cautions
CHLORDIAZEPOXIDE (Rx) **LIBRIUM**	Relieves anxiety and tension; helps control seizures	Drowsiness; slurred speech; weakness; clumsiness	Depression; confusion; excited or agitated behavior; breathing difficulty; liver damage; reduced white-blood-cell counts	This drug can cause psychological and physical addiction even at recommended doses—avoid long-term use. Consult doctor before taking if you are pregnant or are breast feeding. Use caution while driving or operating heavy machinery. Consult doctor before discontinuing this drug after extended use—withdrawal symptoms can occur, including agitation, confusion and seizures.
CHLOROTHIAZIDE (Rx) **DIURIL**	Lowers blood pressure; eliminates fluid	Lightheadedness when standing; increased urination; sensitivity to light; blurred vision; yellow vision	Potassium deficiency; aggravated diabetes and gout; reduced blood-cell counts	Increase intake of potassium-rich foods such as bananas and orange juice. Do not eat licorice, which reduces drug effectiveness. Notify doctor of sore throat, bruising or bleeding—signs of reduced blood-cell counts.
CHLORPROMAZINE (Rx) **PROMAPAR** **THORAZINE**	Controls psychosis; relieves nausea and vomiting	Drowsiness; dry mouth; stuffy nose; difficulty urinating; reduced perspiration; constipation; fast pulse	Reduced white-blood-cell counts; liver damage; impaired vision; stiffness; trembling or twitching; lowered blood pressure; skin rash; severe dizziness	Consult your doctor before taking if you have blood disorders, liver disease, glaucoma, epilepsy, heart disease or lung disease. Inform doctor of sore throat or fever—signs of reduced white-blood-cell counts. Inform doctor if you feel faint, experience heart irregularities or become dizzy, or if you develop yellowing of the whites of the eyes or of the skin—signs of liver damage. Use caution while driving or operating heavy machinery.
CHLORPROPAMIDE (Rx) **DIABINESE**	Controls diabetes mellitus	Diarrhea; nausea; vomiting; appetite loss; headache	Water retention; severe weakness; liver damage; reduced platelet and white-blood-cell counts; lowered blood sugar with overdose	Consult doctor before taking if you have thyroid gland disorders, liver disease, kidney disease, or if you are pregnant or breast feeding. Notify doctor of nervousness, confusion, sweating or weakness—signs of lowered blood sugar. Inform doctor of fever, sore throat, fatigue or unusual bleeding or bruising—signs of reduced blood-cell counts.
CIMETIDINE (Rx) **TAGAMET**	Controls duodenal and peptic ulcers	Diarrhea; dizziness; headache	Behavior disturbances, including confusion and delirium; kidney and liver damage; reduced white-blood-cell count; breast enlargement or soreness	Consult doctor before taking if you have liver or kidney disease, or if you are 60 years of age or older. Take this drug with or just after meals. Take antacids to help relieve stomach pain.
CLOFIBRATE (Rx) **ATROMID-S**	Reduces cholesterol levels in blood	Nausea; diarrhea; stomach pain; weight gain	Irregular heartbeat; chest pain or shortness of breath; reduced white- and red-blood-cell counts; kidney and liver damage; severe muscle pains	Consult doctor before taking if you have kidney or liver disease. Take with food to minimize stomach upset. Consult doctor before discontinuing this drug—stopping abruptly can cause a rebound increase in cholesterol. Inform your doctor of fever, sore throat, bleeding or bruising—signs of reduced blood-cell counts.
CLONAZEPAM (Rx) **CLONOPIN**	Controls epileptic seizures	Drowsiness; slurred speech; weakness; clumsiness	Emotional or behavioral changes; breathing difficulty; liver damage; reduced white-blood-cell count	This drug can cause psychological and physical addiction—use only as directed. Consult your doctor before taking if you are pregnant or are breast feeding. Use caution while driving or operating heavy machinery.

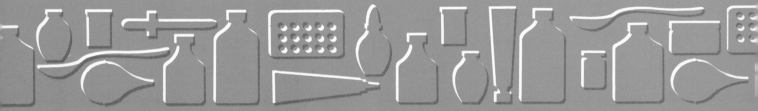

DRUG	Intended effect	Minor side effects	Serious side effects	Special cautions
CLONIDINE (Rx) **CATAPRES**	Lowers blood pressure	Drowsiness; dryness of nose and mouth; constipation; lightheadedness; insomnia; dryness and burning of the eyes	Severe depression; possible congestive heart failure	Do not discontinue drug suddenly—to do so may produce dangerous blood pressure increase. Carry an identification card that states you take this drug; reactions to it are common. Do not take if you have congestive heart failure or heart block. Notify doctor of shortness of breath, a possible symptom of heart failure.
CLORAZEPATE (Rx) **TRANXENE**	Action similar to CHLORDIAZEPOXIDE			
CODEINE, **CODEINE PHOSPHATE** **OR CODEINE SULFATE** **(Rx)** **EMPIRIN WITH** **CODEINE** **TYLENOL WITH** **CODEINE**	Suppresses coughing; relieves mild to moderate pain	Constipation; loss of appetite; upset stomach; drowsiness; skin rash; dizziness	Slowed heartbeat; nervousness; dependence with prolonged use; difficulty breathing; organ damage in victims of kidney, liver, lung or thyroid disease	Consult doctor if you suffer from liver, lung, kidney or thyroid disease, or if you plan to have surgery. Consult doctor if you are pregnant; codeine may affect the function of an embryo or, during labor, impair the breathing of an infant. Drowsiness can make driving or operating heavy machinery dangerous.
CORTISONE (Rx) **CORTONE**	Relieves inflammation	Nausea; indigestion; insomnia; weight gain; muscle cramps; menstrual irregularities	Depression or emotional disturbances; potassium loss; acne; elevated blood pressure; peptic or duodenal ulcer; bone disease; pancreas inflammation; increased pressure in the eye (aggravated glaucoma); impaired immune response	Adhere to a low-salt diet as outlined by your physician. Inform doctor of black tarry stools or persistent stomach pain—signs of bleeding from the stomach or intestine. Do not discontinue abruptly after prolonged use—adverse reactions can occur, such as fever, weakness and dangerous decreases in blood pressure. Do not submit to any vaccinations or skin tests without consulting your doctor.
DEXAMETHASONE **(Rx)** **DECADRON** **DEXONE** **HEXADROL**	Action similar to CORTISONE			
DEXTROMETHOR- **PHAN** **BENYLIN DM** **ROMILAR CF**	Suppresses coughing	Drowsiness; dizziness; upset stomach; vomiting	Difficulty breathing with large doses	Consult doctor if your cough brings up fluid. Drowsiness can make driving or operating heavy machinery dangerous.
DIAZEPAM (Rx) **VALIUM**	Action similar to CHLORDIAZEPOXIDE			
DIGITOXIN (Rx) **CRYSTODIGIN**	Controls heartbeat; increases force of heart contraction	Double or blurred vision; changes in color perception	Severe mental confusion	This drug has a narrow margin of safety; take pills at intervals exactly as prescribed. Carry an identification card that states you take this drug; reactions to it are common.
DIGOXIN (Rx) **LANOXIN** **SK-DIGOXIN**	Action similar to DIGITOXIN			

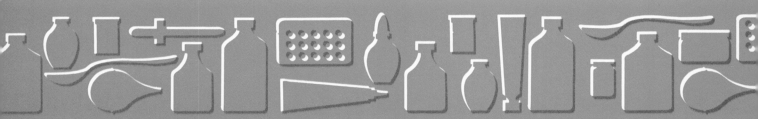

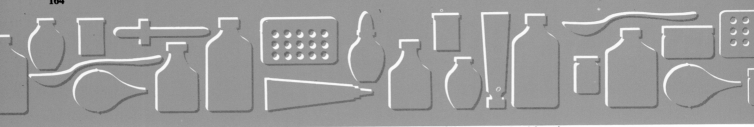

DRUG	Intended effect	Minor side effects	Serious side effects	Special cautions
DIMENHYDRINATE **DRAMAMINE**	Controls motion sickness	Drowsiness; dizziness; dry mouth; nervousness or insomnia, particularly in children	None	Take at least one hour before travel for maximum effect. Use caution while driving or operating heavy machinery.
DIPHENHYDRAMINE (Rx) **BENADRYL**	Relieves allergy symptoms and hay fever; relieves anxiety and insomnia; prevents and controls nausea and vomiting from motion sickness	Drowsiness; dizziness; dry mouth; difficulty urinating	Irregular heartbeat; hallucinations; confusion; delirium; aggravated glaucoma and high blood pressure	Consult doctor before taking if you have glaucoma, high blood pressure, heart disease, or urinary obstruction. Use caution while driving or operating heavy machinery.
DIPHENOXYLATE (Rx) **COLONIL*** **LOMOTIL***	Controls diarrhea and abdominal cramps	Drowsiness; constipation; dizziness; headache	Intestinal obstruction; difficulty breathing with overdose	Consult doctor before taking if you have liver disease or inflammation of the colon (colitis). This drug can cause psychological and physical dependence with extended use in high doses. Use caution while driving or operating heavy machinery. Use with extreme caution in infants and children; they are highly susceptible to side effects.
DISULFIRAM (Rx) **ANTABUSE**	Produces adverse reaction to alcohol—treats alcoholism	Drowsiness; headache; garlicky or metallic taste in mouth	Inflammation of nerves (neuritis); liver damage; psychotic reactions, such as delusions or hallucinations; impaired vision because of optic-nerve damage	Do not take if you have ingested any alcohol in the preceding 12 hours. Avoid all foods, beverages or medications containing alcohol after taking this drug—together the two can produce nausea, vomiting, rapid heartbeat, flushed skin, dizziness, weakness, chest pain, sweating and difficulty breathing. Avoid colognes, liniments or mouthwashes that contain alcohol; absorption of even small amounts of alcohol can cause a severe reaction. Inform doctor of numbness or tingling in hands and feet—signs of neuritis.
DOXEPIN (Rx) **ADAPIN** **SINEQUAN**	Action similar to AMITRIPTYLINE			
DOXYCYCLINE (Rx) **VIBRAMYCIN**	Cures bacterial infection	Nausea; diarrhea; stomach cramps; heartburn; sensitivity to sunlight	Inflammation of the colon (colitis); allergic reactions, such as skin rash, hives, wheezing; reduced red- and white-blood-cell counts; severe headache and blurred vision	Consult doctor before taking if you are pregnant or breast feeding, or if you have any allergies—particularly to any type of penicillin. Avoid use in children under 8 years of age because it can discolor their teeth. Discard unused preparations that are older than 3 months; they can produce kidney damage. Inform doctor if severe diarrhea occurs.
EPHEDRINE **AZMA-AID** **QUIBRON***	Dries and shrinks nasal membranes; relieves asthma	Difficulty urinating; nervousness; insomnia; headache; upset stomach; constipation; loss of appetite; rapid heartbeat; dizziness; feeling of warmth; reduced perspiration	Rise in blood pressure and blood sugar; behavioral disturbances, including confusion, agitation and inappropriate actions; disturbed heart rhythm; aggravated glaucoma	Consult doctor before taking if you have heart or thyroid disease, glaucoma, high blood pressure or diabetes, or if you plan to have surgery in the near future or have difficulty urinating. Do not give to children under 6, or to people 60 or over—groups especially susceptible to disturbed heart rhythm. Reduced perspiration can make exercising or working in hot weather dangerous.

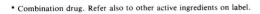

* Combination drug. Refer also to other active ingredients on label.

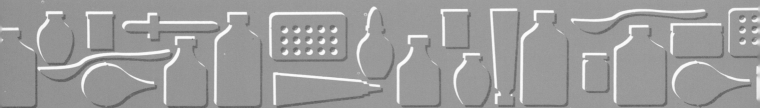

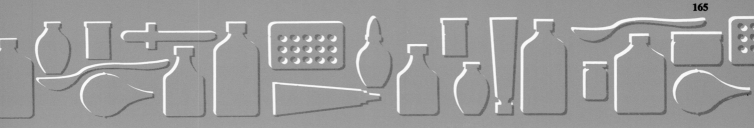

DRUG	Intended effect	Minor side effects	Serious side effects	Special cautions
ERGOTAMINE (Rx) **CAFERGOT** **ERGOMAR**	Relieves migraine headache	Slight tingling or coldness in hands and feet; nausea; dizziness	Chest pain; severe restriction of blood flow to hands, feet or intestines, resulting in tissue death (gangrene)	Consult doctor before taking if you are pregnant or are breast feeding. Inform doctor of red blisters on skin of hands or feet—first signs of gangrene.
ERYTHROMYCIN (Rx) **ERYTHROCIN** **PEDIAZOLE***	Cures bacterial infection	Nausea; vomiting; diarrhea; sore throat; stomach cramping	Liver damage; severe stomach pain; unusual weakness	Take as directed until drug is gone, even if you feel better before your prescription is finished. Inform your doctor if you develop dark urine, abdominal pain, weakness or yellowing of the whites of the eyes or of the skin—signs of liver damage.
ETHINYL ESTRADIOL **ESTINYL** **NORLESTRIN***	Controls menstruation; relieves menopause; in combination with progestin, prevents pregnancy; slows growth of cancer in prostate and breast	Fluid retention; menstrual irregularities; nausea; loss of appetite; breast enlargement or soreness in men and women; diarrhea; skin rash; some loss of scalp hair	Cessation of menstrual bleeding; loss of coordination; pain in legs, indicating blood clots; dangerous rise in blood pressure; cancer in the lining of the uterus	Discontinue and consult doctor immediately if you think you are pregnant. Risk of stroke or heart attack is greater in smokers and in women over 35. Consult your doctor before taking if you have abnormal blood clotting, breast cancer, liver, kidney, gall-bladder or heart disease, asthma, epilepsy or depression.
FENOPROFEN (Rx) **NALFON**	Relieves pain and inflammation	Diarrhea; nausea; dizziness; constipation; dry mouth; headache	Ringing in the ears; severe fluid retention; creation or activation of stomach ulcer; impaired vision; severe skin rash; reduced platelet and white-blood-cell counts; kidney damage	Consult doctor before taking if you have ulcers or have had unusual reactions to aspirin or other drugs used to treat inflammation. Take with milk or food to lessen stomach upset. Use caution while driving or operating heavy machinery. Inform doctor of bloody or black, tarry stools—signs of bleeding from the stomach. Inform doctor of swelling of the legs or feet—signs of excess fluid retention. Inform doctor of sore throat, bruising or bleeding—signs of reduced blood-cell counts. Inform doctor of pain during urination or blood in urine.
FERROUS FUMARATE **FERROUS GLUCONATE** **OR FERROUS SULFATE** **(Rx)** **FERGON** **HEMOCYTE**	Treats anemia by increasing production of red blood cells in the bone marrow	Nausea; appetite loss; constipation; diarrhea	Severe stomach pain; liver damage; shock with overdose	Take with meals to lessen stomach upset. Overdose can cause shock or liver damage in children.
FUROSEMIDE (Rx) **LASIX**	Action similar to CHLOROTHIAZIDE			
GUANETHIDINE (Rx) **ISMELIN**	Lowers blood pressure	Lightheadedness; weakness; blurred vision; nasal congestion; dry mouth; in men, impaired ejaculation	Bone marrow disorder; chest pains; possible congestive heart failure	Notify doctor of sore throat, bleeding or bruising—symptoms of bone marrow disorder. Alcohol, tobacco and carbonated drinks react with this drug. Exercising or working in hot weather may intensify lightheadedness. Notify doctor of shortness of breath, a possible symptom of heart failure.
HYDROCHLORO- **THIAZIDE (Rx)** **ESIDRIX** **HYDRODIURIL**	Action similar to CHLOROTHIAZIDE			

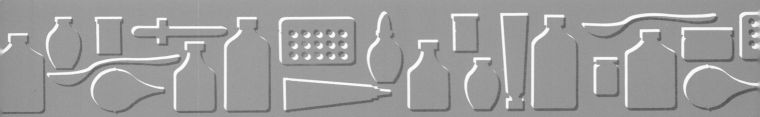

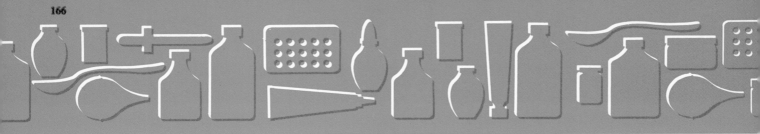

DRUG	Intended effect	Minor side effects	Serious side effects	Special cautions
IBUPROFEN (Rx) **MOTRIN**	Action similar to FENOPROFEN			
IMIPRAMINE (Rx) **JANIMINE** **TOFRANIL**	Action similar to AMITRIPTYLINE			
INDOMETHACIN (Rx) **INDOCIN**	Relieves pain and reduces inflammation	Headache; nausea; vomiting; dizziness	Ringing in the ears; stomach ulcers and bleeding; reduced platelet and white-blood-cell counts; fluid retention; liver damage; blurred vision	Consult doctor before taking if you have liver disease, ulcers or other stomach problems. Take with food or milk to decrease stomach upset. Notify doctor of bloody or black, tarry stools—signs of stomach or intestinal bleeding. Notify doctor of sore throat, bleeding or bruising—signs of reduced blood-cell counts.
LEVODOPA (Rx) **BENDOPA** **DOPAR** **LARODOPA**	Controls symptoms of Parkinson's disease	Diarrhea; constipation; dry mouth; urine discoloration	Lowered blood pressure; irregular heartbeat; behavior changes; uncontrollable movements of the upper body; severe nausea and vomiting	Take with food to reduce stomach upset. Do not drive until you know how this drug affects you. Do not be alarmed if urine discoloration occurs; this is a harmless side effect. Inform doctor of persistent nausea or vomiting. This drug may require several months to produce maximum benefits.
LITHIUM (Rx) **ESKALITH** **LITHONATE**	Controls manic-depression	Thirst; dry mouth; diarrhea	Nausea; vomiting; confusion; weakness; tremors; slurred speech; abnormal thyroid function indicated by swelling in the lower or front part of the neck and thickening of the skin; loss of bladder or rectum control	Take with food to minimize stomach upset. Drink plenty of water while taking this drug—at least 2 quarts daily. Avoid excessive amounts of salt and strenuous exercise in hot weather—may increase side effects.
LORAZEPAM (Rx) **ATIVAN**	Action similar to CHLORDIAZEPOXIDE			
MAGNESIUM **HYDROXIDE** **DELCID*** **DI-GEL*** **GELUSIL***	Neutralizes stomach acid	Diarrhea	Decreased blood pressure; drowsiness; nausea and vomiting—usually in those with kidney disease	Consult doctor before taking if you have kidney disease. Do not take longer than two weeks without consulting doctor.
MAPROTILINE (Rx) **LUDIOMIL**	Action similar to AMITRIPTYLINE			
MESORIDAZINE (Rx) **SERENTIL**	Action similar to CHLORPROMAZINE			
MESTRANOL (Rx) **ENOVID-10** **ORTHO-NOVUM 1*** **OVULEN**	Action similar to ETHINYL ESTRADIOL			

* Combination drug. Refer also to other active ingredients on label.

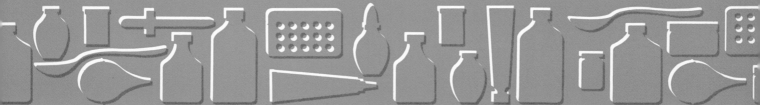

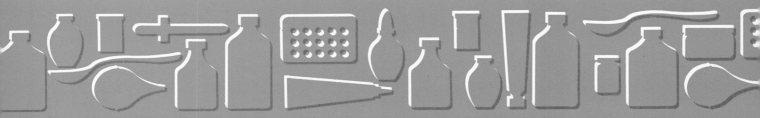

DRUG	Intended effect	Minor side effects	Serious side effects	Special cautions
METOPROLOL TARTRATE (Rx) LOPRESSOR	Lowers blood pressure	Fatigue; overall hair loss; blurred vision	Severe depression; possible congestive heart failure	Do not take if you have heart block or heart failure; it will make these conditions worse. Notify doctor of shortness of breath, a possible symptom of heart failure.
METRONIDAZOLE (Rx) FLAGYL	Cures bacterial and protozoal infections, particularly of the vagina	Diarrhea; nausea; vomiting	Extremely sore mouth or tongue; inflammation of nerves (neuritis); skin rash; reduced white-blood-cell counts	Consult doctor before taking if you are pregnant or are breast feeding. Take as directed until drug is gone, even if you feel better. If you are being treated for a genital infection, recent sexual partners also should be treated. Inform doctor of sore throat or fever—signs of reduced white-blood-cell counts.
MINOCYCLINE (Rx) MINOCIN VECTRIN	Action similar to DOXYCYCLINE			
NALIDIXIC ACID (Rx) NEGGRAM	Cures urinary-tract infections	Nausea; dizziness; diarrhea; itching; rash; vomiting; sensitivity to light	Liver damage; reduced platelet and white-blood-cell counts; blurred, decreased, or double vision, or altered color perception	Consult doctor before taking if you are pregnant or breast feeding. Take with a full glass of water and on an empty stomach. Take as directed until drug is gone, even if you feel better before your prescription is finished. Inform doctor if symptoms worsen or do not improve in a few days. Use caution while driving or operating heavy machinery. Inform doctor of sore throat, bleeding or bruising.
NAPROXEN (Rx) NAPROSYN	Action similar to FENOPROFEN			
NORETHINDRONE (Rx) MICRONOR NOR-Q.D. NORLESTRIN* ORTHO-NOVUM 1*	In combination with an estrogen, prevents pregnancy; slows cancer of the uterus; controls menstruation	Weakness; acne; increased body and facial hair; menstrual irregularities; weight loss or gain; nausea; soreness of breasts; dizziness	Cessation of menstrual bleeding; severe headache; sudden loss of coordination; difficulty breathing; depression	Discontinue and consult your doctor immediately if you think you are pregnant or if you have abnormal vaginal bleeding. Consult your doctor before taking if you have abnormal blood clotting, breast cancer, liver, kidney, gall-bladder or heart disease, asthma, epilepsy or depression.
NORETHYNODREL (Rx) ENOVID*	Action similar to NORETHINDRONE			
OXACILLIN (Rx) PROSTAPHLIN	Action similar to AMOXICILLIN			
OXYPHENBUTAZONE (Rx) OXALID TANDEARIL	Relieves inflammation, principally in arthritis	Nausea; vomiting; diarrhea	Stomach ulcer; kidney damage; impaired vision; reduced white-blood-cell and platelet counts; fluid retention; liver damage	Consult doctor before taking this drug if you have kidney or liver disease, or stomach problems, such as an ulcer. Take with food or milk to lessen stomach upset. Inform doctor of bloody or black, tarry stools—signs of stomach bleeding. Inform doctor of sore throat, bleeding or bruising.
PENICILLIN G AND V (Rx) PENTIDS* V-CILLIN K*	Action similar to AMOXICILLIN			

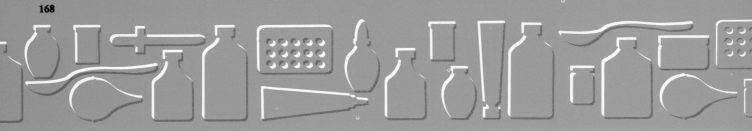

DRUG	Intended effect	Minor side effects	Serious side effects	Special cautions
PENTAZOCINE (Rx) **TALWIN** **COMPOUND***	Relieves moderate pain	Drowsiness; nausea; dizziness; constipation; nightmares	Hallucinations; confusion; difficulty breathing; difficulty urinating	Consult doctor before taking if you have kidney, prostate or respiratory disease. Dependence may occur with prolonged use at high doses. Use caution while driving or operating heavy machinery.
PENTOBARBITAL (Rx) **NEMBUTAL**	Relieves insomnia; relieves anxiety or tension	Dizziness; clumsiness; hangover effect	Difficulty breathing; seizures; confusion; excitement; reduced blood-cell counts; liver damage	Consult doctor before taking if you have lung or liver disease, or if you are pregnant or breast feeding. Dependence may occur with prolonged use at high doses. Do not discontinue abruptly after extended use at high doses—agitation or seizures may occur.
PHENAZOPYRIDINE (Rx) **PYRIDIUM** **UROBIOTIC**	Relieves bladder discomfort and pain	Stomach cramps; dizziness; headache	Lowered red-blood-cell count; kidney or liver damage	This drug imparts a red-orange color to the urine—this is not harmful. Take with meals to lessen stomach upset. Inform doctor of yellowing of the whites of the eyes or of the skin—signs of liver damage.
PHENELZINE (Rx) **NARDIL**	Relieves depression	Dry mouth; constipation; drowsiness; tiredness and weakness; dizziness	Extremely rapid pulse; fainting; severe diarrhea; swelling of legs or feet because of fluid retention; liver damage; severe skin rash; elevated blood pressure	Consult doctor before taking if you have heart, thyroid or liver disease, or severe headaches. Inform doctor of chest pain, vomiting, severe headache or fever—signs of elevated blood pressure. Inform doctor of yellowing of the whites of the eyes or of the skin—signs of liver damage.
PHENOBARBITAL (Rx) **LUMINAL**	Relieves anxiety, tension and insomnia; controls epilepsy	Dizziness; clumsiness; daytime drowsiness or hangover effect when used for insomnia	Difficulty breathing; confusion; excitement; liver damage; reduced blood-cell counts	Consult doctor before taking if you have lung or liver disease, or if you are pregnant or breast feeding. Dependence may occur with prolonged use at high doses. Do not discontinue abruptly after extended use at high doses—withdrawal symptoms, such as agitation and seizures, may occur.
PHENOLPHTHALEIN **ALOPHEN** **EX-LAX** **PHENOLAX**	Relieves constipation	Nausea; diarrhea; pink or red urine; cramping	Allergic reactions, such as skin rash and itching; with prolonged use, severe diarrhea, colic, dehydration and potassium loss	Do not use for longer than one week without a laxative-free period—dependence can occur. Laxative effect may last up to three days. Take on an empty stomach for faster results.
PHENYLBUTAZONE (Rx) **AZOLID** **BUTAZOLIDIN**	Action similar to OXYPHENBUTAZONE			
PHENYTOIN (Rx) **DILANTIN**	Prevents epileptic seizures	Nausea; drowsiness; dizziness; constipation; confusion	Clumsiness; abnormal eye movements and slurring of speech with overdose; bleeding gums; liver damage; reduced red- and white-blood-cell and platelet counts; severe skin rash	Consult doctor before taking if you are pregnant—phenytoin has been associated with increased risk of birth defects. Inform doctor of any signs of toxicity. Inform doctor of weakness, sore throat, bleeding or bruising—signs of reduced blood-cell counts. Do not discontinue use abruptly—may cause severe seizures.

* Combination drug. Refer also to other active ingredients on label.

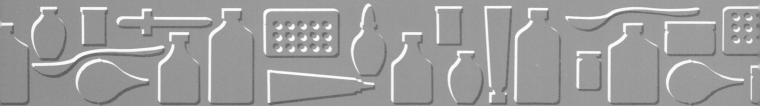

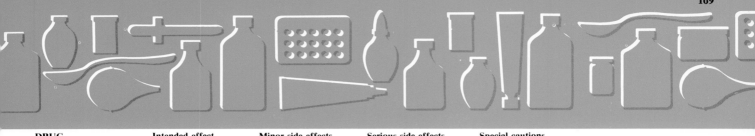

169

DRUG	Intended effect	Minor side effects	Serious side effects	Special cautions
POTASSIUM (Rx) **KAON** **KAY CIEL** **SLOW-K**	Prevents or corrects potassium deficiency, regulating kidney function and conduction of nerve impulses	Nausea; vomiting; diarrhea	Irregular heartbeat; severe weakness; confusion, anxiety; tingling in hands and feet; kidney damage; peptic or duodenal ulcer	Consult doctor before taking this drug if you have kidney disease. Take with food or after meals to minimize stomach upset. Dilute the liquid forms of these drugs with at least 4 oz. of water or juice. Inform doctor of bloody or black, tarry stools—signs of stomach or intestinal bleeding.
PREDNISOLONE (Rx) **DELTA-CORTEF** **HYDELTRA** **STERANE**	Action similar to CORTISONE			
PREDNISONE (Rx) **DELTASONE** **ORASONE** **PARACORT**	Action similar to CORTISONE			
PROBENECID (Rx) **BENEMID**	Reduces uric-acid levels and prevents gout; maintains high levels of penicillin in blood for fighting persistent infection	Nausea; vomiting; appetite loss; dizziness	Kidney stones; allergic reactions, such as skin rash, hives, wheezing, itching; reduced red and white-blood-cell and platelet counts	Consult doctor before taking if you have kidney disease or kidney stones, blood disorders or ulcers. Drink at least five 8-oz. glasses of water to help prevent kidney stones. Inform doctor of weakness, sore throat, fever, unusual bleeding or bruising—signs of reduced blood-cell counts.
PROCHLORPERAZINE (Rx) **COMBID** **COMPAZINE**	Action similar to CHLORPROMAZINE			
PROPANTHELINE (Rx) **PRO-BANTHINE** **ROPANTH**	Relieves spasms and discomfort in digestive tract; treats ulcers	Dizziness; dry mouth; drowsiness; blurred vision; difficulty urinating	Persistent constipation; severe skin rash; increased pressure inside the eye (glaucoma)	Consult doctor before taking if you have colitis, intestinal obstruction, glaucoma or urinary-bladder obstruction. Take 30 minutes before meals unless otherwise directed by your doctor.
PROPOXYPHENE (Rx) **DARVON** **SK-65**	Relieves mild to moderate pain	Drowsiness; dizziness; nausea; constipation	Confusion; difficult breathing; liver damage	Consult doctor before taking if you are pregnant. Dependence may occur with prolonged use at large doses. Use with caution while driving or operating heavy machinery. Inform doctor of yellowing of the whites of the eyes or of the skin—signs of liver damage.
PROPRANOLOL (Rx) **INDERAL**	Controls heartbeat; lowers blood pressure; reduces pain of angina pectoris	Fatigue; cold hands and feet; lightheadedness; overall hair loss	Severe depression; increased risk of asthma; possible congestive heart failure; reduced white-blood-cell and platelet counts	Do not take if you have asthma or hay fever because it increases risk of asthma. Once taking this drug, do not stop suddenly; to do so may cause increased angina or heart attack. Notify doctor of sore throat, bruising or bleeding—signs of reduced blood-cell counts.
PSEUDOEPHEDRINE **NOVAFED** **SUDAFED**	Dries and shrinks nasal membranes	Nervousness; sweating; upset stomach; weakness; insomnia; vomiting; headache; reduced perspiration	Severe behavioral disturbances; elevated blood pressure; slowed heart rate; difficulty urinating	Consult doctor before taking if you plan to have surgery in the near future, if you have difficulty urinating, or if you have heart or thyroid disease, glaucoma, high blood pressure or diabetes. Reduced perspiration can make exercising or working in hot weather dangerous.

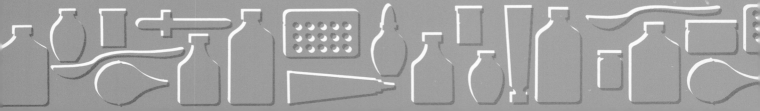

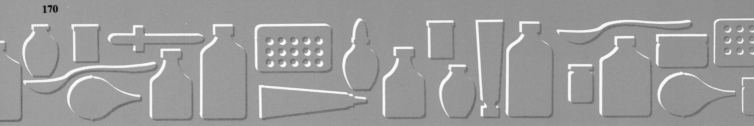

DRUG	Intended effect	Minor side effects	Serious side effects	Special cautions
QUINIDINE (Rx) **QUINAGLUTE** **QUINIDEX** **QUINORA**	Controls heartbeat	Lowered blood pressure; lightheadedness	Fever; reduced white-blood-cell counts	Inform doctor if you have an acute infection of any kind; infection increases possibility of toxic reaction. Carry an identification card that states you take this drug; reactions to it are common. Notify doctor of sore throat, bruising or bleeding—signs of reduced blood-cell counts.
RESERPINE (Rx) **RAU-SED** **SERPASIL**	Lowers blood pressure	Drowsiness; stuffy nose; dry mouth; nausea; diarrhea; appetite loss	Confusion; hallucinations; depression; impotence	Consult doctor before taking if you are pregnant or breast feeding. Inform doctor of signs of depression. Use caution while driving or operating heavy machinery. This drug may take up to 3 weeks to be fully effective.
SECOBARBITAL (Rx) **SECONAL**	Action similar to PENTOBARBITAL			
SULFISOXAZOLE (Rx) **GANTRISIN** **PEDIAZOLE***	Cures urinary-tract infections	Nausea; vomiting; diarrhea	Allergic reactions, such as skin rash, hives, wheezing; muscle aches and pains; reduced blood-cell counts; severe skin reactions; liver damage; kidney damage	Drink plenty of fluids—five 8-oz. glasses of water per day—while taking this medication. Take as directed until drug is gone, even if you feel better before your prescription is finished. Inform doctor if symptoms worsen or do not improve in a few days. Notify doctor of weakness, sore throat or unusual bleeding or bruising—signs of reduced blood-cell counts.
SULINDAC (Rx) **CLINORIL**	Action similar to FENOPROFEN			
TERBUTALINE (Rx) **BRETHINE** **BRICANYL**	Eases breathing in asthma, bronchitis and emphysema	Insomnia; dizziness; nervousness; dry mouth; nausea	Irregular heartbeat; muscle tremors	Consult doctor before taking if you have high blood pressure, heart disease, or diabetes. Notify doctor if difficulty breathing persists.
TETRACYCLINE (Rx) **ACHROMYCIN** **SUMYCIN**	Action similar to DOXYCYCLINE			
THEOPHYLLINE (Rx) **ELIXOPHYLLIN** **SLO-PHYLLIN** **THEO-DUR**	Action similar to AMINOPHYLLINE			
THIORIDAZINE (Rx) **MELLARIL**	Action similar to CHLORPROMAZINE			
THYROID (Rx) **ARMOUR THYROID**	Corrects thyroid hormone deficiency in hypothyroidism; treats thyroid cancer	Allergic reactions, such as skin rash; headache; menstrual irregularities	Irregular heartbeat, nervousness, tremor, vomiting, weight loss, sweating and shortness of breath—signs of overdose; drowsiness, coldness, weakness and weight loss if proper dosage is not maintained	Consult your doctor before taking if you have heart disease, high blood pressure or diabetes. Excessive sweating makes exercise in the heat dangerous.

* Combination drug. Refer also to other active ingredients on label.

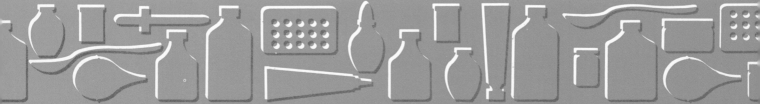

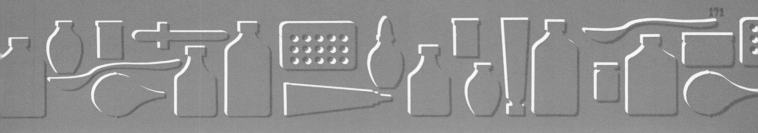

DRUG	Intended effect	Minor side effects	Serious side effects	Special cautions
TOLBUTAMIDE (Rx) **ORINASE**	Action similar to CHLORPROPAMIDE			
TOLMETIN (Rx) **TOLECTIN**	Action similar to FENOPROFEN			
TRIAMCINOLONE (Rx) **ARISTOCORT** **KENACORT**	Action similar to CORTISONE			
TRIFLUOPERAZINE (Rx) **STELAZINE**	Action similar to CHLORPROMAZINE			
TRIMETHOBENZA-MIDE (Rx) **TIGAN**	Relieves nausea and vomiting	Drowsiness; dizziness; drop in blood pressure when given by injection; allergic reactions, such as skin rash; headache	Depression; liver damage; severe trembling and stiffness of arms and legs	Use caution while driving or operating heavy machinery. Inform doctor of yellowing of the whites of the eyes or skin—signs of liver damage.
TRIMETHOPRIM and SULFAMETHOXA-ZOLE (Rx) **BACTRIM** **SEPTRA**	Cures bacterial infection	Nausea; vomiting; diarrhea	Allergic reactions, such as skin rash, hives and wheezing; severe muscle aches and pains; reduced blood-cell counts; severe skin reactions; liver damage; disturbed kidney functions	Drink at least three 8-oz. glasses of water a day while taking this medication. Inform doctor of weakness, sore throat or unusual bleeding or bruising—signs of reduced blood-cell counts.
TRIMIPRAMINE (Rx) **SURMONTIL**	Action similar to IMIPRAMINE			
VALPROIC ACID (Rx) **DEPAKENE**	Controls epileptic seizures	Nausea; vomiting; diarrhea; drowsiness	Liver damage; reduced platelet count	Inform doctor of any unusual bleeding or bruising—signs of decreased platelet count. Inform doctor of yellowing of the whites of the eyes or of the skin—signs of liver damage. Use caution while driving or operating heavy machinery.
WARFARIN (Rx) **COUMADIN** **PANWARFIN**	Prevents blood clots that cause heart attack and stroke	Allergic reactions, such as skin rash, loss of scalp hair or fever; nausea; vomiting; diarrhea	Bleeding	Do not take if you have a tendency to bleed, or suffer from ulcers or ulcerative colitis. Consult doctor before taking if you have high blood pressure, diabetes or a history of liver or kidney disease. Carry an identification card that states you take this drug; it increases severity of accidental bleeding and also reacts with many other drugs. Because drug interactions are numerous, consult doctor before taking any other drug.
ZOMEPIRAC (Rx) **ZOMAX**	Relieves moderate to severe pain; reduces inflammation	Nausea; headache; dizziness; diarrhea; drowsiness; loss of appetite; nervousness	Irregular heartbeat; high blood pressure; urinary-tract infection; vaginitis; depression; liver damage	Use caution while driving or operating heavy machinery.

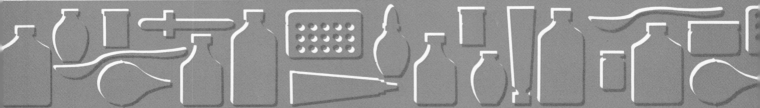

Bibliography

BOOKS

Aikman, Lonnelle, *Nature's Healing Arts: From Folk Medicine to Modern Drugs*. National Geographic Society, 1977.

AMA Drug Evaluations. American Medical Association, 1980.

Berkow, Robert, and John H. Talbott, eds., *The Merck Manual*. Merck Sharpe & Dohme Research Laboratories, 1977.

Burack, Richard, and Fred J. Fox, *The New Handbook of Prescription Drugs*. Random House, 1978.

Clark, W. G., and J. Del Gindice, *Principles of Psychopharmacology*. Academy Press, 1978.

Clarke, Frank H., *How Modern Medicines are Discovered*. Futura Publishing, 1973.

Colton, Theodore, *Statistics in Medicine*. Little, Brown, 1974.

Convictions Under the Food and Drugs Act. American Medical Association, 1917.

Cousins, Norman, *Anatomy of an Illness as Perceived by the Patient*. W. W. Norton, 1979.

DiPalma, Joseph R., *Drill's Pharmacology in Medicine*. McGraw-Hill, 1971.

Dowling, Harry F., *Medicines for Man*. Alfred A. Knopf, 1970.

Drug Topics Redbook 1981. Litton Industries, 1981.

Evaluations of Drug Interactions. American Pharmaceutical Association, 1976.

Florey, H. W., et al., *Antibiotics*. Oxford University Press, 1949.

Garfield, Sol L., and Allen E. Bergin, *Handbook of Psychotherapy Behavior Change: An Empirical Analysis*. John Wiley & Sons, 1978.

Garrison, Fielding H., *History of Medicine*. W. B. Saunders, 1921.

Gerald, Michael C., *Pharmacology*. Prentice-Hall, 1974.

Gilman, Alfred G., et al., *Goodman and Gilman's: The Pharmacological Basis of Therapeutics*. Macmillan, 1980.

Goldstein, Avram, et al., *Principles of Drug Action: The Basis of Pharmacology*. John Wiley & Sons, 1974.

Hansten, Philip D., *Drug Interactions*. Lea & Febiger, 1979.

Haynes, R. Brian, et al., eds., *Compliance in Health Care*. Johns Hopkins University Press, 1979.

The Insight Team of *The Sunday Times* of London, *Suffer the Children: The Story of Thalidomide*. Viking Press, 1979.

Jones, W.H.S., trans. *Hippocrates*. Harvard University Press, 1959.

Kastrup, Erwin K., ed., *Facts and Comparisons, 1981*. Facts and Comparisons, 1980.

Kaul, Pushkar N., and Carl J. Sindermann, eds., *Drugs and Food from the Sea*. The University of Oklahoma, 1978.

Lamy, Peter P., *Prescribing for the Elderly*. PSG Publishing, 1980.

Lasagna, Louis, ed., *Controversies in Therapeutics*. W. B. Saunders, 1980.

Lehrer, Steven, *Explorers of the Body*. Doubleday, 1979.

Levine, Ruth R., *Pharmacology: Drug Actions and Reactions*. Little, Brown, 1978.

Long, James W., *The Essential Guide to Prescription Drugs*. Harper & Row, 1980.

Martin, Eric W., *Hazards of Medication*. J. B. Lippincott, 1978.

The Medicine Show. Consumer Reports Books, 1980.

Mendelsohn, Robert S., *Confessions of a Medical Heretic*. Warner Books, 1979.

Modell, Walter, ed., *Drugs of Choice 1980-1981*. C. V. Mosby, 1980.

Parish, Peter, *The Doctors and Patients Handbook of Medicines and Drugs*. Alfred A. Knopf, 1980.

Physicians' Desk Reference. Litton Industries, 1981.

Physicians' Desk Reference for Nonprescription Drugs. Litton Industries, 1980.

Prescription Drug Industry Fact Book 1980. Pharmaceutical Manufacturers Assoc., 1980.

Robbins, Jack, *Pharmacy: A Profession in Search of a Role*. Navillus Publishing, 1979.

Ross, Walter S., *The Life/Death Ratio*. Readers Digest Press, 1977.

Sandroff, Ronni, ed., *The Potent Placebo*. Litton Industries, 1980.

Sigerist, Henry, *A History of Medicine*. Oxford University Press, 1951.

Sonnedecker, Glenn, *Kremers and Urdang's History of Pharmacy*. J. B. Lippincott, 1976.

Spiegel, Arnold, *The Laboratory Animal in Drug Testing*. Stuttgart: Gustav Fischer Verlag, 1973.

Talalay, Paul, ed., *Drugs in Our Society*. Johns Hopkins University Press, 1964.

Temin, Peter, *Taking Your Medicine*. Harvard University Press, 1980.

United States Pharmacopeia Dispensing Information—1981. United States Pharmacopeial Convention, 1981.

Wardell, William M., ed., *Controlling the Use of Therapeutic Drugs*. American Enterprise Institute for Public Policy Research, 1978.

White, Eugene V., *The Office-Based Family Pharmacist*. Eugene V. White, 1978.

Young, James Harvey, *The Medical Messiahs*. Princeton University Press, 1967.

Young, James Harvey, *The Toadstool Millionaires*. Princeton University Press, 1961.

PERIODICALS

Black, J. W., et al., "Definition and Antagonism of Histamine H_2-Receptors." *Nature*, April 21, 1972.

Brimblecombe, R. W., et al., "Characterization and Development of Cimetidine as a Histamine H_2-Receptor Antagonist." *Gastroenterology*, Vol. 74, No. 2, 1978.

"Continuing Education Courses for Physicians." *JAMA*, Vol. 246, No. 5, August 4, 1981.

"Drugs from the Sea Move Closer to Market." *Chemical Week*, January 28, 1981.

Duncan, William A. M., and Michael E. Parsons, "Reminiscences of the Development of Cimetidine." *Gastroenterology*, Vol. 78, No. 3, 1980.

Faulkner, D. John, "The Search for Drugs from the Sea." *Oceanus*, Vol. 22, No. 2, Summer 1979.

Fink, Joseph L., III, "Physicians' Knowledge of Drug Prices." *Contemporary Pharmacy Practice*, Vol. 1, No. 1, 1978.

Glaser, Martha, "At Last, Unit Sales Take an Upturn." *Drug Topics*, April 17, 1981.

Janssen, Wallace F., "America's First Food and Drug Laws." *FDA Consumer*, June 1975.

Kennedy, Donald, "A Calm Look at 'Drug Lag.' " *JAMA*, Vol. 239, No. 5, January 30, 1978.

Lasagna, Louis, "Placebos." *Scientific American*, Vol. 193, No. 2, August 1955.

"Oral Contraceptives." *Federal Register*, January 31, 1978.

Raloff, Janet, "Drugs That Don't Work." *Science News*, Vol. 119, February 7, 1981.

Ruggieri, George D., "Drugs From the Sea." *Science*, Vol. 194, October 29, 1976.

"The Top 200 Prescription Drugs of 1980." *American Druggist*, February 1981.

OTHER PUBLICATIONS

"Controlled Substances Inventory List." U.S. Department of Justice, Drug Enforcement Administration, January 1979.

"Orphan Drugs and Orphan Diseases, Statement of Lewis A. Engman." Pharmaceutical Manufacturers Association, May 9, 1981.

"Pharmacists for the Future." The American Association of Colleges of Pharmacy, 1975.

Picture credits

The sources for the illustrations that appear in this book are listed below. Credits for the illustrations from left to right are separated by semicolons, from top to bottom by dashes.

Cover: Fil Hunter. 7: John Senzer. 8: From *Art and Pharmacy IV*, Yselpress, Deventer, the Netherlands, courtesy Kunsthistorisches Museum, Vienna. 10, 11: Richard Crist. 13: UPI, King Features Syndicates, Inc., courtesy National Archives (No. 208-LO-9B-28)— King Features Syndicates, Inc., courtesy National Archives (No. 208-LO-9B-10). 15: Henry Groskinsky, courtesy the National Museum of American History—courtesy of the Archives and the Department of Development and Public Affairs, Hahnemann Medical College & Hospital of Philadelphia. 16, 17: Brian Seed. 20: California Primate Research Center, University of California, Davis. 22: Marcia Keegan. 24, 25: Photos courtesy Armour and Company; Enrico Ferorelli. 26: David L. Brill. 27: Photos David L. Brill—John Senzer. 28, 29: Photos Eli Lilly & Co.; Linda Bartlett. 30: Martin Rogers. 31: Photos Martin Rogers—Florita Botts from Nancy Palmer Photo Agency Inc. 32, 33: Photos Eli Lilly & Co. 35: Fil Hunter. 36, 37: State Historical Society of Wisconsin. 39, 40: Library of Congress. 41: Collection of Business Americana, courtesy Smithsonian Institution (Photo No. CBA 5156). 42: Library of Congress. 44: Bayer AG, Leverkusen. 46: Frederic F. Bigio from B-C Graphics. 48: Public Affairs Department, E. R. Squibb & Sons, Inc. 51: Drawing by Karen Karlsson. 53: Fil Hunter. 55: The University Museum, University of Pennsylvania. 60: Leon Dishman, courtesy Walter Reed Institute of Pathology. 61: Drawing by Susan Davis. 64, 65: Fil Hunter. 66: Burt Glinn from Magnum, courtesy Bristol-Myers Co. 68: Eli Lilly & Co. 69: Pfizer Inc. 70, 71: Merck Sharp & Dohme. 72, 73: Eli Lilly & Co., inset, courtesy Warner-Lambert Company. 75: ''The Family Circus'' by Bil Keane © 1979, courtesy The Register and Tribune Syndicate, Inc. 76: Manuscript C-54 Zentralbibliothek, Zurich. 80: Frederic F. Bigio from B-C Graphics. 82: Eli Lilly & Co. 84: George Long for *Sports Illustrated*. 85: Wide World—John Iacono for *Sports Illustrated*. 87: Fil Hunter. 92: Henry Groskinsky, courtesy the National Museum of American History. 93: American Institute of the History of Pharmacy. 94: Henry Groskinsky, courtesy the National Museum of American History. 95: Library of Congress, inset, Henry Groskinsky, courtesy the National Museum of American History. 96, 97: American Institute of the History of Pharmacy—Henry Groskinsky, courtesy The Michael R. Harris Collection; Henry Groskinsky, courtesy the National Museum of American History (2). 98: Henry Groskinsky, courtesy the National Museum of American History. 99: American Institute of the History of Pharmacy—Henry Groskinsky, courtesy the National Museum of American History (2). 100, 101: Library of Congress; Henry Groskinsky, courtesy the National Museum of American History. 103: Fil Hunter. 107: American Institute of the History of Pharmacy. 108: From *Art and Pharmacy II*, Yselpress, Deventer, the Netherlands, courtesy Austrian National Library, Vienna. 109: Photo Bibliothèque Nationale, Paris; from *Art and Pharmacy IV*, Yselpress, Deventer, Holland, courtesy Museum Mr. Simon Van Gijn, Dordrecht, Holland. 110: National Library of Medicine. 113: British Information Services, New York; Library of Congress (2); The Royal Ministry of Foreign Affairs, Press and Cultural Relations Department, Oslo; Greensboro Historical Museum, Inc.—UPI. 116: Yuri Korolev, Moscow. 117: William Campbell from Sygma—Liu Heung Shing, Peking; Masachika Suhara, Tokyo. 118: Courtesy American Pharmaceutical Association. 120-133: John Senzer. 135: Public Affairs Department, E. R. Squibb & Sons, Inc. 137: Mayotte Magnus for *Fortune*. 141: Burroughs Wellcome Co. 142: Merck Sharp & Dohme. 143: Veterinary Resources Branch National Institutes of Health—Merck Sharp & Dohme. 145: American Cyanamid Company. 150: Pfizer Inc. 153-155: © David Doubilet 1977. 156, 157: © David Doubilet 1977; courtesy Phil Alderslade—Dr. F. J. Schmitz, University of Oklahoma. 158, 159: Courtesy Paul D. Shaw; © David Doubilet 1977.

Acknowledgments

The index of this book was prepared by Barbara L. Klein. For their help with this volume, the editors wish to thank the following: I. Asher, Food and Drug Administration (FDA), Washington, D.C.; J. C. Ballin, American Medical Association (AMA), Chicago; E. Barry, FDA, Rockville, Md.; M. Behrman, Health Research Group, Washington, D.C.; D. Berke, Federal Trade Commission (FTC), Washington, D.C.; D. R. Bohardt, American Pharmaceutical Association (APhA), Washington, D.C.; R. Brimblecombe, Smith Kline & French Laboratories, Philadephia; T. Burnett, Tipp City, Ohio; B. E. Byer, FDA, Rockville, Md.; T. E. Byers, FDA, Rockville, Md.; Frank Chappell, AMA, Chicago; R. A. Conrad, Eli Lilly and Company, Indianapolis; J. Controulis, Warner-Lambert Company, Morris Plains, N.J.; L. L. Corrigan, APhA, Washington, D.C.; H. Cothran, FDA, Rockville, Md.; J. Coughlin, AMA, Chicago; D. L. Cowen, Jamesburg, N.J.; A. M. Dozzi, American Society of Hospital Pharmacists, Washington, D.C.; F. Edmonds, National Center for Health Statistics, Washington, D.C.; G. Ennis, Stuart Pharmaceuticals, Wilmington, Del.; N. R. Farnsworth, University of Illinois, Chicago; J. A. Ferguson, National Institute on Drug Abuse, Rockville, Md.; Dr. M. J. Finkel, FDA, Rockville, Md.; J. Forno, Woodstock Colonial Pharmacy, N.Y.; G. N. Francke, APhA, Washington, D.C.; R. Frankel, FDA, Rockville, Md.; L. Geismar, FDA, Rockville, Md.; T. A. Gerding, FDA, Rockville, Md.; V. Glocklin, FDA, Rockville, Md.; Dr. C. Graham, FDA, Rockville, Md.; A. D. Grant, Penick Corporation, Lyndhurst, N.J.; G. B. Griffenhagen, APhA, Washington, D.C.; W. Grigg, FDA, Rockville, Md.; Dr. J. Gwaltney, University of Virginia School of Medicine, Charlottesville; J. A. Halperin, FDA, Rockville, Md.; D. B. Hare, FDA, Rockville, Md.; M. R. Harris, Smithsonian Institution, Washington, D.C.; Dr. M. Hensley, FDA, Rockville, Md.; Dr. R. Hughes, Roswell Park Memorial Institute, Buffalo, N.Y.; R. S. Jacobs, University of California, Santa Barbara; K. W. Johnson, The United States Pharmacopoeial Convention Inc., Rockville, Md.; Dr. J. K. Jones, FDA, Rockville, Md.; S. H. Kalman, APhA, Washington, D.C.; Dr. P. Kaul, Norman, Okla.; Dr. F. O. Kelsey, FDA, Rockville, Md.; G. G. Knapp, FDA, Rockville, Md.; R. Kondratas, Smithsonian Institution, Washington, D.C.; G. G. Koustenis, FDA, Rockville, Md.; R. S. Laderman, FDA, Rockville, Md.; D. Lean, FTC, Washington, D.C.; B. Lee, FDA, Rockville, Md.; M. Lessing, FDA, Rockville, Md.; S. E. Lukas, Johns Hopkins University, Baltimore, Md.; D. V. Lundin, Minneapolis; W. E. Magner, FDA, Rockville, Md.; G. Mallett, Eli Lilly and Company, Indianapolis; J. McElroy, FDA, Rockville, Md.; R. W. McLean, Albany College of Pharmacy, New York; J. E. Moreton, University of Maryland, Baltimore; L. Morris, FDA, Rockville, Md.; A. Mustasa, FDA, Rockville, Md.; D. Naccarto, University of Maryland Hospital, Baltimore; E. Nida, FDA, Rockville, Md.; R. O'Neil, FDA, Rockville, Md.; J. Palmer, Eli

Lilly and Company, Indianapolis; Dr. M. B. Panos, Tipp City, Ohio; R. P. Penna, APhA, Washington, D.C.; M. P. Peskoe, FDA, Rockville, Md.; R. C. Pittenger, Eli Lilly and Company, Indianapolis; M. G. Pleiss, Eli Lilly and Company, Indianapolis; B. Poole, FDA, Rockville, Md.; S. Potkay, National Institute of Health, Bethesda, Md.; Dr. T. E. Prout, American Society of Internal Medicine, Baltimore; W. Purvis, FDA, Rockville, Md.; C. E. Redman, Eli Lilly and Company, Indianapolis; Dr. M. M. Reidenberg, Cornell Medical Center, New York City; T. Reinders, Medical College of Virginia, Richmond; K. L. Rinehart Jr., University of Illinois at Urbana-Champaign; J. Robbins, Schering Laboratories, Kenilworth, N.J.; Dr. E. W.

Rosenberg, University of Tennessee College of Medicine, Memphis; L. Rossiter, National Center for Health Services Research, Hyattsville, Md.; Dr. A. Ruskin, FDA, Rockville, Md.; C. Rutten, FDA, Rockville, Md.; Dr. D. Sackett, McMaster University Health Sciences Center, Hamilton, Ontario; A. C. Sartorelli, Yale University School of Medicine, New Haven, Conn.; F. J. Schmitz, The University of Oklahoma, Norman; C. Schulz, FDA, Rockville, Md.; J. R. Short, FDA, Rockville, Md.; D. H. Shotwell, SmithKline Corporation, Philadelphia; M. Simons, The Proprietary Association, Washington, D.C.; W. E. Small, *American Pharmacy,* Washington, D.C.; D. L. Smith, APhA, Washington, D.C.; R. Solkot, FDA, Rockville, Md.;

G. Sonnedecker, American Institute of History of Pharmacy, Madison, Wis.; W. Storvide, Eli Lilly and Company, Indianapolis; S. A. Stringer, FDA, Rockville, Md.; Dr. R. J. Temple, FDA, Rockville, Md.; D. B. Thomas, Irving, Tex.; Dr. G. Vicik, American Academy of Dermatology, Belleville, Ill.; A. Wachter, SmithKline Corporation, Philadelphia; J. W. Wallace, Merck, Sharp & Dohme, West Point, Pa.; N. Walter, Sterling Drug Inc., New York City; D. M. Ward, Medical Economics Company, Oradell, N.J.; Dr. W. Wardell, Center for the Study of Drug Development, University of Rochester, New York; J. C. Warren, PMA, Washington, D.C.; R. A. Whitney Jr., National Institutes of Health, Bethesda, Md.

Index   *Numerals in italics indicate an illustration of the subject mentioned.*